AF255400

INSOMNIA & OTHER SLEEP DISORDERS:

a comprehensive guide to their causes and treatment

(New Edition)

Dr. Ruth Lever Kidson

Sussex: Sphinx House Publishing

Published by Sphinx House Publishing
East Sussex BN2 8FL

© Ruth Lever Kidson 2014

All rights reserved. No part of this publication may be reproduced in any form or by any means – graphic, electronic or mechanical, including photocopying, recording, taping or information storage and retrieval systems – without the prior permission in writing of the publishers.

The author, Ruth Lever Kidson, has asserted her right under the Copyright, Designs and Patent Act, 1988, to be identified as the author of this work.

This book was originally published in Kindle under the title "Say Goodbye to Sleepless Nights". This new edition (available in Kindle & paperback) has an enlarged section on crystal therapy, a completely new section on circadian rhythm disorders and their treatment, a list of resources, and an index.

ABOUT THE AUTHOR

Dr. Ruth Lever Kidson is a qualified physician, medical hypnotherapist and counsellor, who has trained in several complementary therapies.

She believes that it is important for people to find the treatment that is right for each one personally and that, to this end, they should be given all the information they need to make an informed decision.

This book is an attempt to provide that information so that those suffering from insomnia and other sleep disorders can find it easily in one place.

Other books by Ruth Lever Kidson:

Is Acupuncture Right for You?
Hypnotherapy for Everyone
A Guide to Common Illnesses

PLEASE READ THIS PAGE

Many people with insomnia find self-hypnosis CDs are helpful. Dr. Ruth Lever Kidson has recorded a hypnosis mp3 which is available FREE to readers of this book. You will find the download link in the section on hypnotherapy.

Please note that wherever this image appears in the margin:

it indicates that the section next to it is important and should be read carefully.

CONTENTS

HOW TO USE THIS BOOK

Since you're reading this book, the chances are that you've been plagued by insomnia for some time. You may already have tried various remedies - that you've either read about or that someone else has recommended - and found that they didn't help. And you may even have started to give up hope of finding a cure. So it's important to be aware that your lack of success so far is not because you're resistant to all methods of treatment but simply because you're an individual – you're not a clone of Mr. Brown next door or Mrs. Smith across the street – and what suits other people won't necessarily suit you. It's a question of finding the therapy that's right for you - and the more information you have, the easier that becomes.

In this book I have aimed to tell you as much about as many types of therapy as is possible within a single book of this size.

As you'll see from the list of contents, there's information on eighteen different complementary therapies (and the great variety of remedies available within some of those) as well as an in-depth look at what orthodox medicine has to offer – not just drugs but also behavior therapy and other forms of treatment. And, of course, there's a lot on self-help.

But faced with all this information, you may well be wondering where to start. In order to make the best possible use of this book, what I suggest is this:

 First of all, read the Introduction and Part One. Please don't be tempted to skip this and dive straight into the treatments. Part One contains some very important information about what sleep is and how it can be disturbed. There are many causes of insomnia and, in order to find the most effective form of treatment, it really helps to know *why* you're not sleeping. In addition, there are a number of conditions that masquerade as insomnia, such as obstructive sleep apnea (OSA) or restless legs syndrome (RLS), where the treatment required may be quite different from that for true insomnia.

Once you've read Part One, have a look at the *Do's and don'ts for a good night's sleep* at the beginning of Part Two. Start keeping a sleep journal (as described in this section) and then start to incorporate the suggestions in this section into your lifestyle. At the same time, you could also use the self-help techniques described in the section on *Stimulus control therapy,* and in the sections on *Acupuncture* and *Meditation and visualization.* Give it time. With any long term complaint, you need to be patient because you're not likely to be cured overnight – although I'm not saying that it can't happen! This is where the sleep journal helps – it points up improvements that you might not have been aware of because they happen so gradually.

After a week or two, assess how you're doing. Have the do's and don'ts made a difference? Are you improving? If so, carry on! If, however, the improvement is only slight, you need to decide whether you're going to continue along the self-help route, adding in some of the other methods suggested, or whether you need to see a therapist.

At this stage, you also need to decide whether you should consult your physician, if you haven't already done so. There's a list at the end of Part One telling you when it's essential to have a consultation, but unless you're absolutely certain that you're suffering from primary insomnia or from chronic insomnia resulting from bad habits, you would be well advised to see your physician before starting on any self-help treatments that involve taking remedies or medications. Before you go for your appointment, read the sections on the orthodox treatment of insomnia and (if it seems appropriate) of OSA, RLS and PLMS, and the section on behavior therapy. Then if your physician offers you treatment, you will know what it can (or can't) do and will be able to make an informed decision.

Continuing with the self-help route

Have a look at the other sections that include suggestions on self-help and decide which you like the sound of. Don't try them all at once! The easiest ones to add in at this stage are stimulus control therapy (if you're not already trying it), ayurvedic self-help, shiatsu or yoga.

Once again, see how you go after a week or two. If necessary, change or add another self-help treatment. This may require a trip to the health store to buy aromatherapy oils, flower remedies, herbs, homeopathic remedies or nutritional supplements.

It is most important that you only try these one at a time and that you give them at least a week to ten days to see whether they're making a difference. If there seems to be no improvement with a particular remedy, stop using it before you try something else.

Continue in this way until your journal tells you that there's a definite improvement – and then just carry on with what you're doing until you're cured.

Consulting a therapist

If you decide to see a therapist this will, of course, offer you a choice of several extra therapies which can't be used on a self-help basis. Read through the whole of Part Two and see which therapy appeals to you. When I was practicing as a family doctor, I was frequently aware that, when presented with two or more treatment options, patients tended to have a strong instinct as to which would suit them best. However, if your first choice doesn't have the desired effect, you may find that the therapist who has been treating you will have a clearer idea of which therapy you need.

But whichever route you take – self-help or consulting a practitioner, or a combination of the two – it is vital that you are patient. It's very rare for any therapy, no matter how effective, to work like a magic wand, so you must give it time.

I can't emphasize enough how important this is, particularly if you've suffered from insomnia for a long time.

As the old saying goes "miracles take a little longer". But with patience and perseverance you really should be able to conquer your insomnia and start to sleep well every single night.

INTRODUCTION – WHY IS INSOMNIA SUCH A COMMON PROBLEM?

Human beings are unique in the animal world in that they suffer from insomnia. Cats, dogs, horses, birds . . . they just shut their eyes and go to sleep. But we seem somehow to have lost the knack.

Insomnia nowadays is more common than backache - in fact, it's the third commonest complaint in the US, after headaches and the common cold.

In the US alone, over 70 million people report suffering from insomnia from time to time and about one person in six considers that he or she has a serious sleep problem.

The National Sleep Foundation's *Sleep in America* poll, carried out in 2009, found that only half reported sleeping well every night or almost every night, while a quarter got a good night's sleep only a few times a month or less often. When they were asked about the month immediately past:

- just over 60 per cent of the respondents reported some sort of sleep problem, with two thirds of these saying it had happened every night or almost every night

- just under half of the respondents said that, several times a week, they had spent a lot of the night lying awake and/or had woken up feeling unrefreshed in the morning, while a third had woken early and been unable to get back to sleep and/or had had difficult falling asleep

- about a third had used some sort of "sleep aid" a few times a week

In addition:

- fifteen per cent were using relaxation techniques to help them sleep

- just under one in ten were taking sleep medication prescribed by their doctor

- seven per cent were relying, at least a few nights a week, on alcohol, beer or wine and/or over-the-counter remedies to help them sleep

The report noted that the use of both prescribed sleep medication and over-the-counter sleep aids had increased significantly over the previous few years and that three per cent of insomniacs were using an alternative therapy, such as herbs or melatonin, several times a week.

Millions of dollars are spent each year on sleeping medications, both prescribed and over-the-counter. Insomnia is big business.

So why has this happened and what can be done about it? I hope you will find the answers here. My aim is to offer you unbiased information about the treatments available and how well they work as well as an insight into what causes insomnia, in order to help you get to the root of the problem.

PART ONE – WHY CAN'T I SLEEP?

WHAT IS INSOMNIA – AND HOW MUCH SLEEP DO WE REALLY NEED?

Most people, if asked "what is insomnia?" would reply "not being able to sleep". It seems obvious. But, in fact, there's a lot more to it than that. Doctors include within the definition of insomnia:

- difficulty in falling asleep (sleep onset insomnia)

- waking up frequently during the night and having difficulty getting back to sleep (maintenance insomnia)

- waking early in the morning and being unable to get to sleep again

- waking in the morning feeling that you haven't had enough sleep although you've been in bed for an adequate length of time

- waking in the morning feeling that you've not slept soundly

- feeling unrefreshed after a night's sleep

Some people need considerably less sleep than others in order to function normally – for example, Bill Clinton is said to need only five or six hours and ex-British Prime Minister

Margaret Thatcher needed between four and five. But you don't have to be able to make do with only a few hours in order to be a high flyer – Albert Einstein needed 10 hours a night. It's not the number of hours you sleep but the way you feel afterwards – if you wake feeling refreshed and energetic after only a few hours, you're not suffering from insomnia, you're just very lucky.

However, if you're not one of these fortunate few and you aren't getting enough sleep or you're not getting enough good quality sleep (we'll come to this in the next section) – the symptoms you're likely to suffer from include:

- tiredness (naturally)

- lack of energy

- difficulty concentrating

- irritability

- moodiness

- depression

- poor memory

- decreased ability to solve problems or make decisions

- a greater risk of infections, because adequate sleep is essential for healthy immune system. It has been shown that reducing a person's sleep regularly by two hours a night can result in up to 20 per cent decrease in the white blood cells that combat infections

- you may also find that you're less efficient at work and frequently have to take time off because you don't feel too good after a sleepless night

- and you are also at increased risk of being involved in an automobile accident. Researchers have found that someone who has been awake for 24 hours is as on the ball (or off it!) as someone who has a blood alcohol level of 0.1, which is above the legal limit for driving in most states. It's said that about 70,000 automobile accidents are caused each year in the US by drivers who are drowsy.

TYPES OF SLEEP

Here we get into the scientific stuff. You may be tempted to skip this section and get onto the treatment part – but please don't! In order to be effective, your treatment must be appropriate. And the only way to know what is appropriate is to find out, first of all, what, if anything, is causing your insomnia. And in order to understand that, you need to know something about sleep itself.

Sleep has always been a bit mysterious – why do we need to lapse into unconsciousness for a substantial part of every 24 hours? Over the centuries, various theories have been put forward about the function of dreaming – from shamanic ideas about travelling in dreams and out-of-body experiences, through precognitive dreams (in which we see the future), down to the Freudian belief that dreams are the expression of our subconscious minds. But what of the sleep that produces these dreams? In recent years, scientists have done a lot of research into sleep. And, while they haven't found out why we need to sleep or, indeed, the function of dreams, they have discovered a great deal about the pattern of a normal night's sleep.

There are two types of sleep – REM and NREM. REM stands for "rapid eye movement" and NREM (fairly obviously) for "non-rapid eye movement". REM sleep, in which – as its name implies – the eyes move rapidly under their closed lids, is the form of sleep in which dreams are most vivid and most likely to be remembered.

But the night begins (except in very young babies) with NREM sleep, which is divided into four stages. The changes from one stage into another can be followed by watching an electroencephalogram (EEG) or brain-wave recorder:

- before you even drift into sleep, you have to be in a relaxed state. In this state, the EEG will record so-called alpha waves. Good sleepers will spend less than 10 minutes – and perhaps even only a few seconds - in alpha rhythm before falling asleep. Insomniacs may be here for considerably longer.

- stage 1 – known as light sleep – is what you slip into directly from the alpha state. It's a drowsy transitional state in which your body relaxes, your breathing and your heart rate become slower and the alpha waves are replaced by theta waves on the EEG. Because you're not yet fully asleep, it's easy to be woken from this state.

- the brainwave pattern changes again as you move from stage 1 into stage 2, which is sometimes known as true sleep. Stage 2 is also a light form of sleep, from which it is easy to wake, and if you wake now you may think that you've been awake all along. It has been shown that insomniacs frequently believe that they have slept less than they actually have as a result of waking during stage 2.

- finally you reach deep or slow wave sleep (SWS), so-called because of the slow delta waves recorded by the EEG. This is the deepest form of sleep, in which the body functions are reduced to their lowest level in the 24 hour day. It's very hard to rouse someone from deep sleep because the brain has lost all awareness of the outside world. After about 45 minutes of deep sleep, you have a few minutes more of stage 2 sleep before entering REM.

- REM sleep is sometimes known as paradoxical sleep because, although the body is deeply relaxed and unable to move, the brain is very active and the EEG shows patterns similar to those seen in someone who is fully awake. The heart rate, breathing rate and blood pressure, too, are much the same as they are in the waking state. REM sleep seems to be essential for maintaining emotional balance. People who are deprived of REM sleep may become crabby and bad-tempered. Because alcohol suppresses REM sleep, this is one reason why you can feel so bad after a night of heavy drinking.

The whole sleep cycle from stage 1 to REM takes about 90 minutes and is then repeated four or five times during the night. However, the length of time you spend in each stage changes as the night wears on. The REM section of the first one or two cycles may last no more than a few minutes but lengthens with each cycle, and the last REM of the night may last over an hour. In contrast, the deep sleep stages are longer during the first part of the night. Overall we spend about 5% of each night in stage 1, 50% in stage 2, 20% in deep sleep and 25% in REM.

Whereas newborn babies can sleep up to 20 hours a day and adolescents about nine, most adults find between seven and eight hours adequate and, after the age of 60, this tends to dwindle to around six and a half. The time you spend in the different stages also changes as you get older. Older people spend more time in stage 1 and less in deep sleep than the young and, by the age of 90, deep sleep may have disappeared altogether. As a result, the older you are, the more likely you are to wake during the night. And, because deep sleep is the most restorative form of sleep, older people may feel less refreshed when waking in the morning, even if they have had a relatively good night.

But it's not just age that can affect your sleep patterns. Sudden weight gain or weight loss can disrupt sleep (one reason – among many – why crash diets aren't a good idea). And, of course, jet lag can play havoc with your sleeping patterns for a few days.

In addition, changes in your daily exposure to light and dark may affect your ability to sleep. As light gives way to darkness, the brain starts to secrete a hormone called melatonin which seems to act as a stimulus to sleep. Constant bright light (as has been used in "brain washing") can prevent sleep. On the other hand, complete darkness can disrupt the normal secretion of melatonin and total blindness frequently causes sleep disturbances.

TYPES OF INSOMNIA

At its simplest level, insomnia can be divided into acute (short-term) and chronic (or long-standing) and into primary (without an underlying physical or psychological cause) and secondary (where there is an apparent cause).

Acute or short-term insomnia lasts no more than six months and doesn't occur every night. If it lasts less than a week it is often referred to as transient insomnia.

Transient insomnia is usually due to stress or excitement (as in the Disney World advertisement "I can't sleep, I'm too excited!"), or to noise (the neighbors' kids having a party), to extremes of temperature (being either too hot or too cold), to changes in the sleeping/waking schedule (as occurs with jet lag) or to the side effects of medication.

If you suspect that a medication that you're taking is interfering with your sleep patterns, speak to your physician about it. However, unless the neighbors are whooping it up every night or there's no way to regulate the temperature in your bedroom, this type of insomnia should be easy to deal with.

Chronic insomnia (defined as sleeplessness that has been going on for more than six months or that has occurred almost every night for at least a month) can be more of a problem.

CAUSES OF CHRONIC (LONG TERM) INSOMNIA

The causes of chronic insomnia are numerous but most of them can be grouped into clearly defined categories:

- psychological, psychiatric and emotional

- medical conditions causing pain

- medical conditions causing difficulty breathing

- conditions affecting the body chemistry or the hormone balance

- neurological conditions

- substance abuse and the side effects of medications

- bad habits resulting in acute insomnia becoming chronic

- problems specific to women

- other sleep disorders (which will be dealt with in the next section)

- primary insomnia (where there is no apparent current cause)

Psychological, psychiatric and emotional problems

There must be few people who have never experienced a sleepless night brought on by anticipation of something that is going to happen the following day – whether it's something stressful such as an exam or a funeral or something happy and exciting such as a wedding or a special holiday. But once the event is over, sleeping habits usually return to normal. However, in cases of long-term stress, sleep can be disrupted night after night and chronic insomnia can result.

Sometimes it is anxiety rather than true stress that is responsible. Some people are born worriers and, if this gets out of hand, it needs only the slightest worry – about one's family, one's health or one's job, for example – to cause a sleepless night. And the insomnia then gives another cause for anxiety. So the whole thing becomes a vicious cycle –

anxiety about one's inability to sleep causing insomnia which, in turn, causes more anxiety.

Psychiatric disorders, too, are frequently associated with insomnia. One of the classic symptoms of clinical depression is early morning waking – typically around five or six a.m. – and inability to get to sleep again. Schizophrenia, too, may cause insomnia, as may the manic (or "high") phase of bipolar disorder (manic-depression) when the patient becomes over-excitable and overactive.

Medical conditions causing pain

I saw a cartoon some time ago which showed the inside of a hen-house. Several plump healthy looking hens were sitting dozing on their nests, apparently quite content. But one bird was hanging upside down from a perch saying "I just can't seem to get comfortable". It's a common problem. If we can't sleep, we toss and turn trying to get comfortable. And if we're in pain, it only makes matters worse. Probably the worst culprit is arthritis which, particularly when it affects the shoulders or the neck or the hips, can make it very difficult to get into a comfortable position in order to go to sleep. Fibromyalgia, a condition in which the muscles become painful, can also interfere with sleep. And, of course, even if you do get off to sleep, the pain caused when you move can easily wake you up again.

In most cases where insomnia is due to an underlying medical condition, it is important to treat that condition first because this, by itself, may resolve the insomnia. In the case of chronic pain, this is particularly important since some insomnia treatments may make the underlying medical condition worse. This was particularly so with barbiturates which, thankfully, are rarely used today.

Medical conditions causing difficulty breathing

These include asthma, allergies, lung conditions that may result from smoking (such as emphysema), congestive heart failure and some other heart conditions.

Although sleeping propped up may help the breathing, this is not the most comfortable of positions in which to sleep and so the quality of sleep may not be good.

Conditions affecting the body chemistry

These include kidney disease, which results in waste products being inadequately cleared from the blood stream, and hormonal disorders such as hyperthyroidism.

Neurological disorders

Patients who suffer from Parkinson's disease may have difficulty sleeping. Paradoxically, people with chronic fatigue syndrome may also suffer from insomnia. Tinnitus, a constant ringing in the ears caused by degeneration of the nerves involved in hearing, can keep someone awake just as easily as any other constant noise.

The side effects of medications and substance abuse [1]

Overindulgence in **alcohol** or the use of "recreational" drugs can cause insomnia, as can an excessive intake of caffeine.

Insomnia is a recognized side effect of **beta-blockers** (prescribed for a variety of conditions including high blood pressure, angina and other heart problems including abnormal rhythms, and as a preventive treatment for migraine), **clonidine** (used to treat high blood pressure), **theophylline** (a treatment for asthma and chronic bronchitis), some types of **antidepressants**, some **steroid** preparations, **decongestants**, **stimulants** and pain killers that contain **caffeine**,.

Beta-blockers may be prescribed under their generic or their trade names and include:
acebutolol (Sectral)
atenolol (Tenormin)
betaxolol (Kerlone)
bisoprolol (Zebeta, Cardicor, Emcor, Monocor)
carteolol (Cartrol)
carvedilol (Coreg)
celiprolol (Celectol)
esmolol (Brevibloc)
labetalol (Normodyne, Trandate)
metoprolol (Lopressor/Lopresor, Toprol, Betaloc)
nadolol (Corgard)
nebivolol (Nebilet)

---

1 Please note that, where orthodox drugs are discussed in the text, the generic name is given together with one or two of the trade names. Some drugs appear under a variety of names in different countries and no claim is made here to include them all.

oxprenolol (Trasicor)
penbutolol (Levatol)
pindolol (Visken)
propranolol (Inderal)
sotalol (Betapace, Sotacor, Beta-Cardone)
timolol (Blocadren, Moducren, Betim)

Clonidine is marketed under the trade names of Clorpres, Combipres or Catapres and, in the UK, as Dixarit which is approved for the treatment of migraine and menopausal hot flashes.

Theophylline is found under a large variety of trade names including Franol & Nuelin.

The **antidepressants** that may affect one's sleeping habits are SSRIs (selective serotonin reuptake inhibitors) and the older, and now less commonly used, MAOIs (monoamine oxidase inhibitors). Both can cause increased waking during the night. SSRIs include:

       citalopram (Cipramil, Celexa)
       escitalopram (Lexapro, Cipralex)
       fluoxetine (Prozac)
       fluvoxamine (Luvox, Faverin)
       paroxetine (Paxil, Asimia, Seroxat)
       sertraline (Zoloft, Lustral).

MAOIs include:

       isocarboxazid (Marplan)
       moclobemide (Aurorix, Manerix)
       phenelzine sulfate (Nardil)
       tranylcypromine sulfate (Parnate).

Another MAOI, selegiline (Eldepryl, Zelapar) is used only to treat Parkinson's disease.

Corticosteroids, which are sometimes used to treat asthma and painful inflammatory conditions such as rheumatoid arthritis, may be a cause of insomnia. They include:

> betamathazone (Betnelan, Betnesol)
> deflazacort (Calcort)
> dexamethazone (Decadron)
> fludrocortisone (Florinef)
> hydrocortisone (Hydrocortone)
> methylprednisolone (Econopred, Medrone)
> triamcinolone (Azmacort, Nasacort).

These steroids are also commonly prescribed in the form of creams for the treatment of inflammatory skin conditions. However, because such creams should be used sparingly and for a short time only, it is highly unlikely that enough will be absorbed into the system to cause generalized side effects such as insomnia.

A number of **pain killers**, including over-the-counter preparations, contain **caffeine**. These include Migril and Cafergot (both of which are specifically designed for the treatment of migraine), Anacin, Excedrin, Genaced, Propain, Resolve Extra, Syndol, Vanquish, Veganin and Wigraine.

Most **decongestant** preparations (either prescribed or over-the-counter) contain ephedrine or pseudoephedrine which can cause insomnia.

Therapeutically, **stimulants** are usually prescribed to treat narcolepsy or attention deficit hyperactivity disorder in children and adolescents. The active ingredients are methylphenidate (for example, in Concerta, Focalin and Ritalin) and dexamphetamine.

Bad habits that turn acute (short term) insomnia into chronic insomnia

These will be dealt with more fully in the section on behavioral therapy. Suffice it to say here that it's all too easy, after a few bad nights resulting from an acute problem (perhaps anxiety relating to a specific event or incident) for someone to become anxious about the insomnia and set up a vicious cycle which then becomes difficult to break.

Why women suffer from insomnia

Women are twice as likely to suffer from insomnia as men. During their reproductive years, the fluctuating hormone levels associated with the menstrual cycle and with pregnancy may disrupt their normal bodily rhythms and may also make them more vulnerable to emotional stress.

Symptoms of the premenstrual syndrome may include difficulty in getting to sleep, waking during the night and, as a result, increased sleepiness during the day.

Pregnant women may find that they sleep well during the first trimester (first 12 weeks) and may also be sleepy during the day. But by the third trimester, the need to pass water because of pressure on the bladder, heartburn, fetal movements, low back pain, leg cramps and nightmares may all combine to make it very hard to get a good night's sleep.

Around the menopause, sleep problems tend to become more frequent. Insomnia may be associated with depression due to the change in hormone levels, while hot flashes and night sweats may result in disturbed nights.

Primary insomnia – insomnia without a cause

When all possible underlying causes have been ruled out, a diagnosis of primary insomnia can be made. If the problem started in childhood without any precipitating upset or trauma, it may be classified as idiopathic, particularly if it's associated with hyperactivity or attention deficit disorder. But for most people it's due to tension and habit.

Usually it begins with a prolonged period of stress. Most of us have had the odd sleepless night worrying about our work or a member of our family or how we're going to pay a large bill, or any one of a number of other reasons why we get anxious and stressed. But once the anxiety is resolved, the majority of us revert to our former sleeping patterns. Some people, however, remain sleepless. Over time, as the insomnia shows no signs of abating, their previous anxiety is replaced by an anxiety about sleeping and, instead of going to bed in a relaxed frame of mind, they become increasingly tense as bedtime draws closer.

Almost invariably, people with this sort of insomnia are perfectly able to fall asleep when they don't want to, such as while they're watching TV or sitting in meetings. They may become obsessive about the problem to such an extent that their thoughts and their conversations increasingly revolve around the subject and it comes to the point where it seriously affects their quality of life. They try hard to sleep, but this only results in their making themselves more tense. Their pre-bed routine, such as brushing their teeth, emptying the trash and checking that the doors are locked, may start to generate tension and they begin to dread going to bed. However, away from their normal environment – staying in a hotel or with friends, for example – they are able to sleep perfectly well.

OTHER CAUSES OF DISTURBED SLEEP

Snoring

We tend to think that the only people who suffer as a result of snoring are those who have to lie awake listening to it, while the snorer sleeps on, oblivious to the disturbance he (or she) is causing. But snoring is a symptom of sleep disordered breathing (SDB) which includes a range of conditions in which the upper part of the airway (in the nose and throat) is obstructed, the most severe form being obstructive sleep apnea (OSA).

Snoring occurs as a result of vibrations set up when air can't pass freely through the nasal passages and throat. It doesn't happen when we're awake because our natural muscle tone prevents it, but once we're asleep these muscles relax and, if there's any form of obstruction in the air passages, snoring will result.

There are quite a number of physical factors that can cause snoring. These include being overweight (fat deposits in your neck which cause a double chin may, when you lie down, obstruct your throat), nasal congestion (due to a cold or an allergy), nasal polyps and an over-large soft palate. Other factors include smoking (the smoke can cause irritation and swelling of the lining of the airways), drinking alcohol (which encourages the muscles to relax even more than they normally would during sleep), breathing through your mouth, and sleeping on your back (because this allows the tongue to drop back and partially obstruct the throat). In women, both pregnancy and the menopause may herald the onset of snoring although, in pregnancy, it may be transient.

Although the snorer may not realize it, the fact that he snores – and therefore doesn't breathe normally – during the night may result in him feeling tired during the day, having a poor memory and difficulty concentrating. Women who snore are likely to suffer from these symptoms as well but, in addition, are more likely to complain of depression and insomnia. In order to find the right treatment, therefore, it is important to know whether a woman presenting with either of these problems is a snorer.

Obstructive sleep apnea (OSA)

Obstructive sleep apnea is one of a group of conditions, known as Sleep Disordered Breathing (SDB), in which the upper part of the airway (in the nose and throat) becomes partially or even completely blocked during sleep, preventing the free flow of air into and out of the lungs. It is believed to affect one man in 25 and one woman in 50, although the incidence is higher in obese people. It is also more common in African-Americans and in Indian men than in Caucasians.

It is estimated that only around one tenth of people with OSA seek treatment, the main reason for this being that sufferers do not recognize the condition for what it is. They believe that the reason they are tired during the day is because they wake up a lot during the night, and they just label this as insomnia. But the reason they wake is because, at frequent intervals throughout the night, the upper airway collapses in on itself, forming a block and they stop breathing, usually for a period of 10 to 30 seconds. This results in sufferers waking up, partly or fully, sometimes gasping for air. They may thrash around during the night, talk in their sleep or even sleepwalk. Other symptoms include profuse sweating, heartburn, headaches and a dry mouth the following morning, and even bedwetting. In all cases, when morning comes, they will not feel fully rested or refreshed.

OSA is commoner in men than in women and about one third of affected men will also suffer from lack of libido, impotence and ejaculatory problems. In addition, sufferers may complain of depression, memory impairment and problems maintaining relationships. There is also evidence that untreated sleep apnea may increase the risk of developing high blood pressure, heart problems and insulin resistant diabetes.

Because patients with OSA are usually not aware of what is happening – other than that their nights are disturbed – it may be necessary for them to spend a night or two being observed in a sleep laboratory in order for the diagnosis to be made.

Parasomnia

Parasomnia is a 'catchall' term which covers all sleep disorders that involve abnormal movement, behavior, perceptions, emotions and dreams that occur when we're sleeping, falling asleep or waking up . . . things such as sleepwalking, grinding our teeth, confusion on waking, twitching our legs, or talking in our sleep.

What actually causes any of these things is not known. However, what is known is that, for some people, they can be brought on by stress, drinking alcohol, lack of sleep, fever, physical exertion, depression, and certain medications. Several are more common in children than in adults. However, **REM Sleep Behavior Disorder**, in which the sleepers act out their dreams, is most commonly seen in adult males and may sometimes be a side effect of antidepressants.

Of course, the danger in REM Sleep Behavior Disorder, and in **sleepwalking,** is that the sleepers will harm themselves or others. However, not all parasomnias have this problem and some, such as **catathrenia**, in which the sleeper takes a deep breath, holds it and then lets it out slowly, often with a loud groan or squeal, are just a nuisance – primarily for whoever is sleeping in the same room.

Teeth grinding (bruxism), is irritating to listen to and also can, in the long term, put wear on the teeth and, in some cases, cause pain in the jaw. **Hypnagogic hallucinations** and **sleep paralysis**, however, have no long term effects but can be quite scary. Hypnagogic hallucinations are dreams, which may be frightening and which occur just as the person is falling asleep. They may cause the sleeper to wake with a sudden jerk. Sleep paralysis happens just as the person is waking. This usually occurs immediately after a dream, and the inability to move which is normal during dreams persists for a few minutes after waking.

Each parasomnia has its own appropriate treatment and anyone who is exhibiting symptoms of any of these conditions should consult a physician.

Restless legs syndrome (RLS)

Unlike those with OSA, patients with restless legs syndrome are all too aware of what troubles them. Towards the end of the day they start to develop unpleasant sensations in their legs – described in many cases as pins and needles and "internal" itching or a crawling sensation. These sensations become worse when they lie down in bed and are relieved only by moving. As a result, they have great difficulty falling asleep.

The condition can begin at any age but tends to be mild before middle age. Indeed, it's not uncommon for it to remain undiagnosed for ten or twenty years after its onset. But in about two thirds of patients the symptoms get gradually worse and, in some cases, may become intolerable. Some patients also have unpleasant sensations in their arms or elsewhere on their body.

The diagnosis is made simply on the symptoms that are reported by the patient – an urge to move the limbs, associated with unpleasant sensations, restlessness (such as tossing and turning in bed or constantly rubbing the legs), the symptoms being worse at rest and in the evening and night and being eased by movement.

RLS can run in families and is made worse by fatigue, stress, extreme heat or cold, caffeine, tricyclic antidepressants and drug withdrawal. It sometimes seems to occur as a result of kidney failure, polyneuropathy (a deterioration of the nerve endings which is occasionally due to alcohol abuse), diabetes, rheumatoid arthritis, or anemia which may be due to a deficiency of vitamin B12 (pernicious anemia), iron or folic acid. Between 25 and 40 per cent of pregnant women develop RLS but it usually disappears within a few weeks of the birth of the baby.

About 85 per cent of patients with RLS also suffer from periodic limb movement in sleep (PLMS), which is sometimes called nocturnal myoclonus.

Periodic limb movement in sleep (PLMS)
Like snoring, this is a condition that can disturb the patient's bed partner while the patient remains quite

unaware of it. Common over the age of 65, PLMS consists of repetitive jerks of the legs and (less frequently) the arms, occurring every 20 to 60 seconds. Very often this will rouse the patient but not to a degree where he or she is aware of it. The only symptoms tend to be feeling unrefreshed by the night's sleep and being sleepy during the day.

Sometimes PLMS occurs in patients with kidney or liver failure, OSA or narcolepsy and may result from drug withdrawal states. It can also be a side effect of certain medications, including the tricyclic antidepressants. These include:

> amitryptiline (Elavil, Endep, Tryptizol)
> amoxapine (Asendin [US], Asendis [UK])
> clomipramine (Anafranil)
> doxepin (Sinequan)
> imipramine (Tofranil)
> lofepramine (Gamanil)
> nortriptyline (Allegron, Aventyl, Pamelor)
> trimipramine (Surmontil).

Night terrors (sleep terrors)

When a sleeper wakes suddenly in the night, screaming, sweating and with a racing pulse, this may be an episode of night terrors. The condition is seen most often in children (where it can affect up to one in fifteen) but becomes progressively uncommon with age and is very rare over the age of 65.

Usually, sufferers will sit up in bed, often with eyes wide open even though they're still asleep. They may lash out (this is more common in adults) or even get out of bed and run around. It's difficult to wake them and, once awake, they tend to be confused. Some may remember a fragment of a terrifying dream, a few may remember a complete dream, but others remember nothing at all. Some people experience episodes only a few times a year but others have them more frequently – in severe cases they may occur almost every night. However, they rarely occur more than once in a single night.

Unlike nightmares, which happen in the REM cycle of sleep (after you have been asleep for 90 minutes or so), night terrors occur earlier, usually within the first hour of sleep. And by the time the morning comes, the sufferer may have no recollection of the event at all.

Night terrors may begin when a child is three or even younger, but they tend to diminish and die out during the teenage years. Very often they run in families and may be associated with sleepwalking and talking in the sleep.

Although the cause of night terrors is not understood, it is known that certain things may precipitate an episode. These include lack of sleep, PMS, stress, travelling, alcohol, eating a large meal late at night and, in children, fevers. Because some of these (such as lack of sleep, alcohol intake and eating late) can be regulated, it is possible for the sufferer to control the attacks to some extent. Obstructive sleep apnea (OSA) can also make night terrors worse.

Narcolepsy

The common perception of narcolepsy is that it causes sudden lapses into deep sleep, even in the middle of activity. But in some instances it may be hard to distinguish from insomnia. This is because, in mild cases, a narcolepsy sufferer may complain simply of disturbed sleep and feeling very tired and sleepy during the day.

However, narcolepsy is very much less common than insomnia, affecting only one person in every 2000, and in many cases it is accompanied by other symptoms. If there is any doubt, it can be diagnosed by measuring the brainwaves of the sleeping patient.

Narcolepsy is thought to be an auto-immune disorder – a condition in which the body's defenses turn upon parts of the body itself. (The commonest of these conditions is rheumatoid arthritis). In narcolepsy, there is evidence that this causes a reduction in a certain protein, hypocretin, in the brain. Since hypocretin plays an important role in regulating sleep patterns, sleep disturbances result when the levels are inadequate.

The main difference between narcolepsy and insomnia is that the narcoleptic patient will feel very tired and sleepy even after a good night's sleep. Another difference is that, with normal sleep, some 90 minutes or so will pass before dreaming begins. But narcoleptic people will dream within ten minutes of falling asleep. However, like insomniacs, narcolepsy sufferers may also have disturbed nights, with frequent waking.

Other symptoms that may occur include transient muscle weakness (which can often be brought on by laughter, anger or other emotions), sleep paralysis (occurring just before sleeping or else on waking, where the person is unable to move, sometimes for up to 30 minutes), and hallucinations that, like sleep paralysis, can occur when going into or coming out of sleep. These three symptoms – weakness, sleep paralysis and so-called hypnagogic hallucinations – together with excessive sleepiness during the day form the classic symptoms of narcolepsy. However, the four only occur together in about 25 per cent of sufferers – and while the sleepiness is something that will continue throughout life, the other symptoms may disappear in time.

CIRCADIAN RHYTHM (OR BODY-CLOCK) DISORDERS

Most people who have done long-haul flights will have suffered from a circadian rhythm disorder - commonly referred to as 'jet lag'. It's when your body and the clocks around you don't agree on what the time is. Fortunately, jet lag is a temporary condition which can be cured by a few nights' good sleep.

However, for some people, their body clocks seem to be always out of synch. These circadian rhythm disorders are rare but I have included this section for two reasons: firstly because they are often misdiagnosed as a more common sleep disorder (and therefore incorrectly treated) and, secondly, because recent advances in drug therapy may mean that it will be easier to treat them than it was in the past. (Treatment for these disorders is discussed in the 'Orthodox Treatment' section.)

Delayed Sleep Phase Disorder (DSPD)

People who suffer from this condition often can't fall asleep until well after midnight and then have great difficulty waking at a 'normal' hour. If it's possible for them to keep their own hours (for example, going to bed at 2am and sleeping through till 10am) they have no problems, will sleep well and won't feel tired until the early hours of the following morning.

DSPD usually develops in childhood or adolescence and parents may struggle to get affected children to go to bed and stay there. However, if the children are allowed to stay up until they feel sleepy, they will sleep normally once they are put to bed. If the condition arises in adolescence, it may prove to be temporary, disappearing in early adulthood but, for other sufferers, it's permanent. Sedatives taken at night aren't helpful because, while they may produce relaxation and even a feeling of tiredness, they won't induce sleep.

Some people with DSPD have, of necessity, to work a 9 to 5 day but this may result in symptoms such as fatigue, headaches and depression unless they're able to sleep on into the afternoon at weekends.

DSPD is an uncommon condition, affecting about 3 people in every 2000. However, there is a much higher rate in adolescents, with the vast majority being boys, although there are equal numbers of men and women among adult sufferers.

Unfortunately, DSPD is often misdiagnosed. Parents, teachers and employers may think that the sufferer is just lazy. Where a doctor has been consulted, other diagnoses, such as depression, may be made, resulting in inappropriate medication.

Advanced Sleep Phase Disorder (ASPD)

This rare condition tends to run in families and affects men and women equally. Sufferers start to feel sleepy very early in the evening and wake very early. If they go to bed when their bodies tell them that they need to, they will sleep normally and not have any symptoms during the day. However, if they force themselves to stay up to a later hour, they will still wake at their usual time so that they are likely to develop all the symptoms that go with lack of sleep.

Irregular Sleep Wake Rhythm

This is a rare condition in which sleep patterns are completely irregular. Sufferers will take numerous naps during the course of 24 hours, but these will all be of short duration, with no prolonged period of sleep either at night or during the day, although the total amount of sleep is likely to be normal for their age. The sleep pattern will vary from day to day and, because the quality of sleep may be poor, patients may feel very tired much of the time.

Non 24 Hour Sleep Wake Disorder (N24HSWD) or Hypernychthemeral Syndrome)

N24HSWD mainly affects people who are totally blind. This is because light helps to control our circadian rhythms by regulating the body's secretion of the hormones melatonin and cortisol, both of which play an important role in our waking-sleeping pattern. For people who are totally blind, this regulation is lost and, while not all of them suffer from N24HSWD, it's been estimated that it affects at least 70%. However, for reasons which are less clear, it can also affect sighted people, although this is very rare. But because the symptoms are often not reported to a doctor or are misdiagnosed as a type of insomnia, the true figures are unknown.

The symptoms can be very similar to those of insomnia - disturbed sleep at night, associated with fatigue and sleepiness during the day, together with problems with memory and concentration, and even depression.

Because in blind people the production and suppression of hormone secretion is not affected by light, the normal 24 hour circadian cycle may be extended. For example, if someone has a cycle of 24½ hours, if he goes to sleep at ten o'clock one night, the following night he is unlikely to be able to sleep before 10.30. and, by the end of the week, he will be lying awake until 1.30 in the morning. After another two weeks, he will feel wide awake all night and ready for sleep at 8.30 in the morning. Eventually he will start to sleep at night again, but the extended rhythm will continue so that, while he has some periods when he can sleep well at night, there will be others when it's impossible.

If N24HSWD develops in a totally blind person, it usually does so quite soon after all sight has been lost. Some people try to cope by forcing themselves to go to bed and get up at the same times as they have always done. However, this is likely to result in extreme symptoms of fatigue which may be misdiagnosed as depression, chronic fatigue syndrome or a form of insomnia.

All circadian rhythm disorders are rare and many doctors are unaware of them. If you think you or someone you know may be suffering from N24HSWD, I recommend that you consult these two websites which can advise you on how to how to talk to your doctor about the problem:
http://sleepfoundation.org/non-24/facts_prevalence.html
http://www.non-24.com/

END OF PART ONE

BUT BEFORE YOU GO ON TO THE NEXT SECTION . . .

The next section will describe in detail what can be done about insomnia with the help of orthodox, complementary and self-help treatments. However, **you should consult your physician before starting to use any form of complementary or self-help treatment if you fall into any of the following categories:**

- you are taking medications prescribed by your physician

- you are kept awake by pain

- you have difficulty breathing

- you are a heavy drinker

- you take "recreational" drugs

- you are suffering from depression

- you snore loudly or have any reason to believe that you may be suffering from obstructive sleep apnea

- you have any form of kidney or liver disease or any other chronic illness

 In addition, **you need to ensure that any complementary therapist you consult is qualified to treat you.** Phone and ask where he[2*] trained and for how long and whether he has malpractice insurance. A properly qualified practitioner will never mind being asked these questions.

---

*   Throughout this book I refer to physicians and therapists as "he". I apologize if this offends anyone but to keep repeating "he or she" is cumbersome and to use "they" is ungrammatical. Perhaps in a couple of hundred years the English language will have evolved and there will be an all-encompassing word for both genders!

PART TWO – WHAT CAN I DO?

DO'S AND DON'TS FOR A GOOD NIGHT'S SLEEP

In order to find the best treatment for your insomnia, it's important to try to find out what's causing it. However, no matter what the cause, there are certain self-help measures that are well worth trying. A lot of them are just plain common sense and may be things that you do already. And some are ideas that you might not have thought of. Try those that seem to be appropriate to your own case. They may take time to work, so it's important not to be impatient. But you should start to see some improvement within a few weeks.

However, whichever method or methods you decide on, you should, in addition, keep a sleep journal. Begin this before trying any form of therapy, be it orthodox drug treatment, behavioral therapy, complementary therapy or even self-help and continue to keep it until you're sure that your sleeping patterns are steadily improving. Every morning, record in your journal what time you went to bed the previous night, approximately how long it took you to fall asleep, how many times you woke during the night and roughly how long it took you to get back to sleep again and, finally, how you felt in the morning.

Not only will this help you to understand your insomnia and the reasons why certain therapies might be more suitable for you than others, but it will also give you a record of how your treatment is progressing. So, if the weeks go by and you find yourself thinking "this is hopeless, I still wake up in the night and lie awake for hours", you can go to your journal and find, for example, that, although you woke up twice last night and it took you perhaps fifteen minutes to get back to sleep again, three weeks ago you woke four times and took up to half an hour to fall asleep. Curing insomnia is a gradual process and it's important not to get discouraged!

One important point, though – when you record in your journal the length of time it took you to fall asleep, this should be an approximation. If you keep looking at the clock to check the time, that in itself will help to keep you awake!

Things to avoid

Although the title of this section is "do's and don't" it's easier to take them in the order of "don'ts and do's". So here are the things to avoid:

- **caffeine**: try to limit your caffeine intake, especially in the hours before bedtime. Remember that it's not just coffee that contains caffeine – there's caffeine in tea, in chocolate and in cola. The effect of caffeine is to speed up the brainwaves (whereas, as we've seen, sleep is associated with a slowing down of brainwaves), increase the heart rate and the blood pressure, increase alertness and reduce tiredness. It can also make you want to urinate during the night, disturbing your sleep by making you have to get out of bed. It works within 15 minutes and can last for over six hours, which is something to consider when you're deciding what's the latest you can drink a cup of coffee. If you're particularly susceptible, you may want to restrict yourself to decaff tea or coffee or, better still, fruit or herb teas in the late afternoon and evening, and may even want to avoid eating dark chocolate at night.

Some people seem not to be affected by caffeine and so don't have to worry about this – as with all these measures, if it doesn't help, don't do it (but give it a few weeks before deciding that it doesn't).

- **alcohol**: avoid drinking more than 1 fluid ounce of alcohol during the evening. Although alcohol depresses the brain so that it's easier to get to sleep, it makes sleep lighter and more fragmented because it suppresses both deep (or slow wave) sleep and REM sleep. If you've had a few drinks the night before, you're more likely to wake in the morning feeling unrefreshed, even if you didn't drink enough to have a hangover. Alcohol should always be avoided in the evening by people with obstructive sleep apnea (OSA) because it relaxes the muscles of the throat even more and so can make the condition worse.

- **smoking**: if you can't give up smoking completely, try not to smoke in the evening. The effects of nicotine are similar to those of caffeine – it speeds up the brain waves, the heart rate and the breathing rate and affects the body in much the same way that stress does. And the effects can last for several hours after smoking one cigarette. A number of studies have shown that, when smokers give up, they sleep better even though they may have temporary withdrawal symptoms such as restlessness and anxiety, which tend to last about 10 days. Once the withdrawal symptoms have gone, sleep improves even more.

If you're in the process of giving up smoking, you may be using nicotine patches to help you. The instructions usually tell you to remove the patch at bedtime but, if you're not sleeping well, you may find that removing it an hour or two before you go to bed will help you sleep better.

- **cat naps**: don't nap during the day if you can possibly help it, as this may result in your being less sleepy at bedtime. If you really can't do without a nap, take it in the early afternoon and for no more than 30 minutes. Alternatively, you could try the system practiced in many hot countries of having a proper siesta of two hours after lunch, in which case you would expect to sleep correspondingly less at night. However, if you do this, you must do it every day. Having a siesta once or twice a week will disrupt your sleeping patterns even more.

- **heavy meals**: avoid heavy meals late at night. Your whole body needs to be resting when you lie down in bed – including your stomach.

- **hunger**: avoid going to bed hungry. You won't get to sleep if your stomach's rumbling. However, if you do need a snack before bedtime, avoid sweet things because these will raise your blood sugar and this may stop you falling asleep.

- **strenuous exercise**: avoid strenuous exercise in the evening. We'll go into the reason for this in the "things to do" section.

- **television**: avoid watching television just before you go to bed. Do something restful, such as listening to music or meditating (more about this later on).

- **clock watching**: once you're in bed, don't watch the clock. Thinking "Oh good grief, it's one thirty and I'm still not asleep," does nothing to put you into the relaxed frame of mind you're trying to achieve. And if your clock has a loud tick, either move it well away from the bed or buy another one that's quieter.

- **light**: if you need to get up in the night to go to the john, don't put the light on. If you can't manage in the dark, buy a night-light that you can plug into a socket in the hallway – it'll give you enough light to stop you stumbling around but not enough to wake you up fully.

OK, that's the don'ts. So what *should* we do? The "do's" fall into three groups – lifestyle changes, things to do before bedtime and things to do once you're in bed.

Lifestyle changes

- **learn to reduce or manage stress**. Yes, I know – much easier said than done. But there are ways – meditation, yoga, biofeedback and others. We'll talk more about meditation and yoga later on. If you tend to worry about little things, a simple method of reducing anxiety is to spend time in the early evening making a list of everything you're worrying about – and then write down what you can do about each of them.

- **exercise regularly**. In order to sleep well, our bodies need to be relatively cool. Body temperature rises during exercise but, a few hours later, it will drop significantly to compensate and this persists for up to four hours, making it easier to fall asleep and to stay asleep. But if you exercise within three hours of bedtime you could still be too warm when you go to bed (you may not even be aware of this) and it may prevent you from falling asleep.

Exercise also has a tranquilizing effect which has been shown to last at least four hours and to be more effective in reducing anxiety than many anti-anxiety medications. It can work in mild or moderate depression, as well – one study compared exercise with the antidepressant Zoloft and found that they were equally effective, while another found that patients reported feeling better within a week of starting an exercise program.

Researchers at the Stanford University School of

Medicine looked at the effects of exercise on a group of sedentary adults aged between 55 and 75 who were complaining of insomnia. The participants exercised for 20 to 30 minutes every other afternoon – doing aerobics, walking or riding a stationary bicycle – and the time they needed to fall asleep was reduced by half, while the time they slept was increased by almost an hour.

Before bedtime

- **have a warm milk drink**. The calcium it contains is a muscle relaxant, while another constituent is converted by the body into a substance which prompts the brain to produce the chemical serotonin. And one of the actions of serotonin is to make you feel sleepy. However, the drink has to be warm – cold milk doesn't have the same effect.

- **try relaxing with soft music, meditation or a warm bath**. But because the bath will raise your body temperature, don't take it within two hours of going to bed.

- **turn down the lights**. If we lived entirely by natural light, when dusk fell our brains would be stimulated to produce a chemical called melatonin whose effect is to lower our body temperature and make us feel sleepy. Although electric light is not nearly as bright as sunlight, a strong light can still inhibit the production of melatonin.

By changing the times when you are exposed to bright light, you can change your sleeping patterns. So people who have difficulty getting to sleep may find that getting out in the sunshine early in the morning, which will cause their body temperature to rise and fall earlier in the day, may help them to fall asleep more readily. On the other hand, people who wake up too early in the morning may find that some bright light in the early evening will change the rhythm of the rise and fall of their body temperature so that they will sleep longer. They may, however, find that they don't get off to sleep as easily as before. If you find that a change of exposure to light is helpful, it may be worth buying a light box or some daylight spectrum light-bulbs to ensure that you get adequate light during the winter months. (Using these bulbs around your home is also helpful if you suffer from winter depression or SAD – Seasonal Affective Disorder.)

In recent years it has been shown that blue light makes us more wakeful, whereas pink light is soothing. This seems to be something that human beings developed long before there were electric lights, when it was important to wake up with the dawn and go to sleep at sunset. (This, of course, is something that many animals and birds still do automatically.) There is quite a lot of blue in ordinary light bulbs but it's now possible to buy special bulbs that cut out the blue component. Television, too, is a powerful source of blue light, but you can buy special tinted spectacles which will filter out the blue coming at you from the screen.

- if you're feeling hungry when it's coming up to bedtime, **have a light snack** of some turkey, tuna, bananas, figs, dates, yogurt, or peanut butter – all of which contain the amino acid L-tryptophan which helps to promote sleep. There is also tryptophan in milk.

Bedtime

- **go to bed and get up at the same time every day**. Obviously this won't always be possible if you want any sort of social life, but try to get into a regular routine. Having said that, don't go to bed until you're sleepy. So when you're deciding on your routine, choose a time at which you tend to start feeling drowsy.

- **make sure that your room is well ventilated and neither too hot nor too cold.** If your body temperature is too high you'll have difficulty falling asleep and, because your deep sleep will be reduced, you'll be more likely to wake during the night. But it's also difficult to sleep if you're cold. If you tend to get cold in the night, try wearing socks in bed – there is some evidence that if your feet are warm, the rest of your body will stay warm too.

- **keep light and noise to a minimum in the bedroom**. If it doesn't trouble you, have heavy drapes to shut out the light. If you suffer from claustrophobia, you may find this oppressive, so try using an eye-mask – it will block out the light but is less likely to make you feel shut in. As far as noise is concerned, we can't always control it. But there are very good earplugs on the market that are comfortable to wear and really work – ask at your local drugstore. If you prefer, you could buy a sound conditioner – a gadget that produces a continuous noise that sounds like flowing water or falling rain which has the effect not only of blocking out other noises but of relaxing the brain and so making sleep easier. And, as I've already said – if your bedside clock has a loud tick, get a quieter one.

- once you're in bed, **don't read, eat, chat, make 'phone calls or watch television**. Use the bedroom only for sex and for sleep. That way, the mind gets to associate it with sleep and not with activity (well, apart from the sex!). However, although sex is an 'active sport', the body's response to it is to feel drowsy afterwards, so it may well help you to sleep.

- whether or not you sleep, **don't stay in bed for longer than eight hours**. We shall return to these last two instructions when we look at behavior therapy.

And finally, TRY NOT TO WORRY ABOUT NOT SLEEPING. This is not easy when you've had a succession of sleepless nights. But the trouble is, the more you worry about not being able to sleep, the worse the insomnia is likely to become. If you can, just allow yourself to accept the fact that you're not sleeping well – for the moment – and remain positive in the knowledge that, in due course, things will get better.

A NOTE ABOUT MEMORY FOAM

A lot of claims have been made for memory foam pillows and mattresses - not only that they will promote restful sleep but also that they can relieve migraine and other painful conditions such as sciatica, can prevent pressure sores in people who are bed- or chair-bound, and can reduce the frequency of asthma attacks. As a result, sales have climbed steadily since memory foam came onto the market nearly twenty years ago.

Known technically as visco-elastic polyurethane foam, memory foam moulds itself to the shape of the person lying on it. So, unlike a standard mattress, it supports but doesn't rub or press on tender parts of the body. This means that sleeping on memory foam should be more comfortable and should, to some extent, reduce tossing and turning in the night since this is usually in response to discomfort.

The foam is responsive to the heat of the body and holds that heat. So, while this may be an advantage when it is used as a pillow to alleviate neck or shoulder pain, some people may find that they get uncomfortably hot at night when lying on memory foam. And, unfortunately, when it gets damp (if the heat causes excess sweating), the foam tends to retain the moisture. However, different degrees of foam density are available and the less dense varieties allow greater airflow which keeps them cooler than the more dense type.

Because memory foam supports the body more evenly than a traditional mattress and so can be very helpful for people suffering from painful back problems and fibromyalgia where distortion of the body as may occur during sleep can increase the pain.

Different experts have different opinions on memory foam. Some suggest that you will find instant comfort on a foam mattress while others believe that it can take several weeks to get used to. Some say that asthma attacks may be reduced by sleeping on a memory foam mattress which others point out that, while a denser foam may have this effect (because house dust mites, to which asthma sufferers are often allergic, find it hard to get a hold in it), there is little difference in this respect between the more open foam and traditional mattresses.

Some recommend a density of 4lb as the ideal for most people, while others suggest anything between 4 and 6lb. Similarly, some believe that the best depth of foam is between 3 and 5 inches, whereas others say that more than 3 inches may reduce rather than increase the level of comfort.

Memory foam is not cheap so, with all these varying opinions, it's important to make sure you're getting exactly what you need when you buy a mattress or pillows. Getting as much advice as you can before buying is important. The thing to remember is that not all memory foam is the same but, if you find out which type is right for you, you are likely to increase your comfort and be able to sleep better as a result.

SIMPLE STRATEGIES FOR SPECIFIC CONDITIONS

Simple strategies for the treatment of PLMS and RLS

There is considerable overlap in the treatments for these two disorders. Both can be made worse by caffeine, alcohol and nicotine, so these should be avoided or, if that's not possible, intake should be reduced to a minimum. If you're taking medication of any sort, check with your physician as to whether it might be contributing to the problem (some anticonvulsants, antidepressants and tablets for high blood pressure can have this effect). If it is, your physician may be able to change your prescription.

If you have a vitamin B12 deficiency or an iron deficiency (both of which can be checked with a blood test), these need to be corrected. If iron is prescribed (usually in the form of ferrous sulfate) it should be taken together with vitamin C about an hour before a meal, in order to increase absorption.

Simple physical therapies may also be helpful – gentle exercise, whirlpool baths, leg massage or using a vibrator (on the feet!) before bedtime. If you have varicose veins, wearing support hose will help to keep them in check and prevent your legs from feeling heavy.

Simple strategies for the treatment of snoring and OSA

Treatment of snoring should begin with simple self-help methods:

- If you are overweight, losing some weight should help. However, the body needs carbohydrates in the diet in order to produce the chemical serotonin which is important for the maintenance of our sleeping patterns. So a diet which dramatically reduces your carbohydrate intake (such as the Atkins diet), while helping you to stop snoring, may interfere with your sleep in other ways. Perhaps the best diet around at the moment is the low GL diet, which is easy to follow and well-balanced.

- Cut down or stop smoking

- Anything that may make the over-relaxed throat muscles relax still further should be avoided. This includes sleeping tablets, sedatives and, in the evening, alcohol.

- Make a conscious effort to sleep on your side. Sometimes tipping up the head of the bed can be helpful but you should only use one pillow because more than this will cause your chin to sink onto your chest and increase the obstruction in your throat. You may find that a pillow which is designed to help you sleep on your side is useful. Or you can try wearing a bra back-to-front with tennis balls in the cups!. Sleeping on your side allows your tongue to drop forward and to the side, so that it doesn't block the airway.

- If you have allergies which cause nasal obstruction,

these should be treated and you should ensure that you have hypoallergenic pillows.

- If you tend to be a mouth breather, adhesive strips, which are designed to keep your mouth closed during the night and encourage nasal breathing, may help.

- There are sprays available whose astringent properties will help to minimize any swelling in the lining of the air passages.

- A recent piece of research showed that, in a survey of over 800 professional musicians, those who played double-reed woodwind instruments, such as the bassoon and the oboe, had a lower risk of OSA than those who played other instruments. This suggests that the breathing techniques involved in playing these instruments can train the throat muscles to remain firm, even in sleep. Of course, to be a professional musician, requires long hours of practice but it is possible that even playing a double reed instrument as an amateur could, as long as the practice was regular, be beneficial.

OVER THE COUNTER MEDICATIONS

The sort of sleep medication that you can buy over the counter can be divided into two main groups – the 'orthodox' (that is, drug-based – in most cases, an antihistamine) and the complementary - mainly herbal preparations and nutritional supplements).

Most over-the-counter herbal remedies for insomnia contain valerian, which is discussed in the section on herbs. Other preparations that are used induce sleep are tryptophan, 5-HTP and melatonin, all of which are discussed in the section on Nutrition Therapy and Supplements.

The main use of antihistamines is in the treatment of allergies. They do induce sleepiness but they can have unpleasant side effects, too. You may find that your mouth is very dry or your vision is blurred. Taken regularly, they can also cause disturbances of the digestive system – either constipation or diarrhea. They can make asthma worse and so should never be taken by anyone who suffers from asthma. And this type of medication should also be avoided by pregnant women and those who are breast feeding, as it might affect the baby.

END OF PART TWO

PART THREE – WHAT CAN MY DOCTOR DO? - ORTHODOX TREATMENTS

PRESCRIBED MEDICATIONS

For centuries people have searched for the perfect sleeping drug, or hypnotic, to give it its proper name. And for the past fifty or sixty years, they have searched – not entirely successfully – for drugs that would be safer and less likely to be addictive than those which they already had.

During the nineteenth century, opium based medications were used as everyday sedatives. Laudanum was very popular and many people became addicted. Non-opium hypnotics included chloral hydrate (first manufactured in 1832) and paraldehyde. However, both of these were very unpleasant to take and could have nasty side effects. In the early twentieth century barbiturates were discovered and produced in huge numbers. As with laudanum, their capacity to cause addiction was not recognized and many people, once on them, found it impossible to come off again. In addition, barbiturates were very dangerous in overdose, particularly if taken with alcohol, and became a common way of committing suicide.

Addiction and safety are the two major problems confronting those who seek to find drugs that will tranquilize or sedate the human brain. In the 1960s and early 1970s a new "wonder drug" was introduced – methaqualone (Mandrax). It was believed to be safe and non-addictive and was widely prescribed for insomniacs and also, to a lesser degree, for patients suffering from anxiety and high blood pressure. However, it became clear after some years that it was, in fact, highly addictive and, as a result, was banned.

Unfortunately, the experience of Mandrax was not an isolated episode. It may take some years before doctors become aware that a new drug is addictive and even longer before the investigations to confirm this are complete. In 2002, twelve years after it had first been introduced, the United States Food and Drug Administration (FDA) published a warning that the widely used and supposedly safe antidepressant paroxetine (Paxil, Seroxat) could produce severe withdrawal symptoms in some patients who tried to stop taking it. And, of course, it took a considerable time before people became aware that the benzodiazepines which used to be extremely popular both as sedatives and as hypnotics - drugs such as diazepam (Valium), temazepam (Restoril) and lorazepam (Ativan) – could cause dependency and withdrawal effects when the drug was stopped.

It's little wonder, therefore, that more and more people are becoming nervous about taking drugs of any sort. However, there is no doubt that, in certain diseases and conditions, some drugs can be life-saving or can greatly improve the patient's sense of well-being and so the only thing that you can do is to be guided by health professionals and by common sense. In an emergency life-threatening situation, we are forced, by necessity, to accept the treatment which is likely to be most effective, whether that treatment will have side effects or not. However, with less dramatic conditions, a balance needs to be struck between what is most effective and what is safest. Sometimes they are the same, in which case there is no problem. In other cases, however, a decision needs to be made after very careful thought.

The current thinking among medical practitioners is that sleeping tablets should only be prescribed in the short term, even though the modern generation of drugs appears to be far safer and less addictive than previous types.

Here I want to emphasize once again that if you know or suspect that your insomnia is due to an underlying medical or psychiatric condition – whether it be arthritis, asthma, depression or any of the other conditions listed in the section on causes of insomnia – you must consult a physician. Although treatment of the underlying condition doesn't always cure the insomnia, it may well improve your sleeping pattern and, certainly, if you leave the condition untreated and only try to treat the insomnia, the chances of anything working are small.

Once the diagnosis has been confirmed and orthodox treatment offered, it is up to you whether you decide to take it or to try complementary methods. Obviously this will depend on the condition itself. If you are suffering from an overactive thyroid, for example, it would be advisable to accept orthodox treatment whereas, if you have arthritis, you might feel that acupuncture or homeopathy offers you a better balance of effectiveness with safety.

If you are quite certain that the reason for your insomnia is neither medical nor psychiatric, you need to try to see what the real reason is. Are you under stress? Do you do shift work? Are you being disturbed by noise or excessive light or by a restless bed partner? Did you have a few bad nights (for whatever reason) and then start worrying that you couldn't sleep and so get into a vicious cycle? Or have you developed what the health professionals call "poor sleep hygiene" – in other words do you go to bed at a different time every night and, when you get there, read the newspaper, listen to the radio, drink cups of tea, do crosswords – in other words, have you done everything possible to make your subconscious mind stop associating the bedroom with rest and relaxation?

I'm not suggesting that if your insomnia has no underlying medical or psychiatric cause, you should consider taking sleeping tablets, any more than I would suggest that, if there is a known cause, you should not. In some cases treatment of the underlying cause *plus* a short burst of sleeping tablets may be helpful. Where there is no cause, certainly a few weeks of tablets may help to break a vicious cycle, but it may be that there are better methods of treatment.

So, supposing that you go to see your physician and he recommends that you take some medication, what is it likely to be? Whatever he gives you, it is unlikely to be for more than a few weeks and he may advise you to take it for only two or three nights every week. You will probably be started on a low dose and asked to report back on its effectiveness. If it's not working well, the dose can be increased until the optimum is found. Your physician may also recommend that you have some behavioral therapy, which we will discuss later. If you are suffering from depression, he may suggest an anti-depressant which has sedative properties, rather than a sleeping tablet. And, as we shall see later on in this section, anti-depressants may also have a role to play in the treatment of elderly people with insomnia.

Hypnotics vary according to how quickly they act and for how long. Those with a rapid onset of action are used to treat patients who have difficulty falling asleep, while those which take longer to be eliminated from the body and therefore act over a longer period of time are more suitable for people who tend to wake up during the night. However, hypnotics which are eliminated very slowly can cause daytime sedation and so tend to be avoided.

Ultimately, whether or not to take sleeping pills must be a personal choice, with guidance from a medical professional. Understanding the drawbacks, as well as the advantages, of the proposed drugs will help you to make an informed choice as to whether, for you, sleeping pills will be helpful or not.

Benzodiazepines (BZDs)

Although benzodiazepines are no longer as popular as they used to be (as a result of increased awareness of the risk of dependency and withdrawal effects), they are still prescribed and are, indeed, useful for some patients. It is as well, however, to be aware of their drawbacks:

- they are unsafe in pregnancy

- the longer acting varieties, such as flurazepam (Dalmane) are unsuitable for elderly people because the fact that they are eliminated more slowly in the elderly may lead to a cumulative effect resulting in sleepiness during the day, lethargy, an inability to think clearly, unsteadiness and an increasing risk of falling

- if they are stopped suddenly, insomnia may follow that is worse than before they were started (so-called "rebound insomnia")

- they may also cause anxiety if you suddenly stop taking them

- if used every night, or nearly every night, they will lose their effectiveness. It is estimated that, after using them every night for about three to four weeks, most benzodiazepines become no more effective than a placebo.

- although they increase the total amount of sleep, this is lighter than normal because they suppress deep sleep and REM sleep.

- they can produce a hangover effect that makes it harder to think clearly than after a sleepless night.

Americans spend more than $400 million on benzodiazepines every year and a good proportion of them have been taking these drugs for a long time. In the United Kingdom, the National Institute for Clinical Excellence has estimated that between 10 and 30 percent of long-term benzodiazepine users are physically dependent on them (in other words, addicted), and that 50 percent of all users have withdrawal symptoms when they come off them. Withdrawal can be a prolonged affair and can start at any time up to three weeks after stopping a long-acting preparation or within a few hours of stopping a short-acting one. The symptoms include anxiety, depression, nausea and, as mentioned above, rebound insomnia.

So why should anyone ever want to take benzodiazepines? Well, for a start, because they work and, in the short term, can be very useful. In addition, while you continue to take them, they reduce anxiety and so, for patients who are suffering from anxiety as well as insomnia, they can kill two birds with one stone.

There are several benzodiazepines that are commonly used to treat insomnia. Some are licensed in some countries but not others. Some, such as triazolam, have been withdrawn in certain countries where they were once available while remaining available in others.

The reason why there is a variety of BZDs on the market for the treatment of insomnia is that they vary according to how long they remain in the blood stream (and therefore how long they remain active). For someone who has difficulty getting to sleep (sleep onset insomnia), a short acting drug may be all that is needed, while someone who regularly wakes during the night and has difficulty getting to sleep again (sleep maintenance insomnia) may need an intermediate or longer-acting formulation. In addition, while most BZDs work to counteract anxiety, some are better than others and this needs to be taken into consideration if anxiety is playing a large part in the patient's insomnia.

Among the best known benzodiazepines (listed with some, but not all, of their trade names) are the following:

- temazepam (Restoril, Temaze, Euhypnos) which has an intermediate action and is used for both sleep onset insomnia and sleep maintenance insomnia; it can be useful when the insomnia is severe

- lorazepam (Ativan, Tavor, Temesta) which is a powerful intermediate-acting (sleep maintenance) drug and is particularly useful when there is associate severe anxiety

- oxazepam (Serax, Seresta) and estazolam (ProSom) which are intermediate acting and are used for sleep maintenance insomnia

- flurazepam (Dalmane, Dalmadorm) which is long-acting and can stay in the blood stream for up to four days. This means that some people who take it will find that it makes them feel excessively sleepy during the day, so it is not suitable for everybody. It tends to be used for sleep onset insomnia and sleep maintenance insomnia that is mild or moderate

- quazepam (Doral), like flurazepam, is long-acting and can be used for both sleep onset insomnia and sleep maintenance insomnia. However, tests have shown that it is better than other BZDs in that it has fewer side effects, is less likely to cause rebound insomnia when it's stopped and is less likely to lose its effectiveness with continued use.

- midazolam (Dormicum, Hypnovel) is a short-acting BZD which is used for moderately severe sleep onset insomnia in patients who haven't been helped by other drugs

- lormetazepam (Noctamid, Dilamet, Sedaben) and loprazolam (Dormonoct, Sonin, Somnovit) are used to treat moderately severe sleep onset insomnia and sleep maintenance insomnia. Lormetazepam is not licensed in the USA.

- flunitrazepam (Rohypnol) has gained notoriety as the 'date rape' drug. In some countries it is regulated as a narcotic. However, it does have a use in the treatment of severe chronic insomnia that has not responded to other medications.

Temazepam and oxazepam are also used in the treatment of anxiety.

Because they all belong to the same family of drugs, the benzodiazepines all tend to have the same contraindications and side effects. So, for example, most or all are contraindicated for patients with the eye condition known as narrow angle glaucoma, for patients with untreated obstructive sleep apnea (because they can make it worse by relaxing the throat muscles still further), for those who have a history of substance abuse (because of the risk of addiction) and for pregnant women. They are also not advisable for patients with depression (because they may depress the mood still further), liver or kidney disorders (because they may not be adequately broken down and excreted from the body) or lung complaints (because they may depress the breathing). And in almost all cases they will be prescribed only for a limited period of time – sometimes for just a week or two.

The commonest side effects include drowsiness during the day, dizziness, difficulty thinking clearly, unsteadiness with an increased risk of falls (especially in the elderly), and rebound insomnia and other withdrawal symptoms when they are stopped. Patients taking triazolam have sometimes complained of loss of memory.

In order to reduce the risk of withdrawal symptoms and rebound insomnia, it is essential that benzodiazepines are never stopped suddenly. They have to be tapered off – for example, if you've been taking them every night, you will need to reduce the dose to every other night, then to every third night, then every fifth night and finally to once a week before stopping completely. The length of time over which this tailing-off should be done will depend on which benzodiazepine you've been taking, whether it's short or intermediate or long-acting, and also on how long you've been on the tablets, but in all cases will be over a number of weeks. This is something about which your physician will advise you.

The "Z drugs" – zaleplon, zolpidem and zolpiclone

The latest generation of sleeping pills is made up of the so-called "Z drugs" - zaleplon (Sonata), zolpidem (Ambien) and zolpiclone (Zimovane). They are said to have fewer side effects than benzodiazepines but, even so, shouldn't be taken by people who have untreated OSA or a history of substance abuse and should be avoided by patients with liver or kidney disease. Very short term treatment is normally recommended (not more than two to three weeks) since longer treatment can result in dependence followed by withdrawal effects once the drugs are stopped, although it is possible to take them over a longer period if they're only used on two or three nights a week. And, again like the benzodiazepines, the Z drugs should be tapered off rather than stopped abruptly, in order to reduce the risk of rebound insomnia.

There is the possibility, particularly in the elderly, that the Z drugs can cause lack of co-ordination and unsteadiness, difficulty thinking clearly or nightmares and, if the tablets are stopped suddenly, hallucinations may occur. These side effects only occur in a small percentage of patients but it's important to realize that, although they may be safer than benzodiazepines, the Z drugs are not risk free.

However, to break the vicious cycle of insomnia causing anxiety causing insomnia, a short course of one of the Z drugs may be all that's needed. Similarly, in cases where the patient says (justifiably) "I know I'd feel so much better if only I could get a good night's sleep", a short course may result in a much greater ability to cope with whatever circumstances have been causing the insomnia.

But, in many cases, a course of pills – for however long a period of time – will just be papering over the cracks. In such cases, sleeping tablets can be either replaced by or combined with another therapy.

Ramelteon

An even more recent development is ramelteon (which is marketed under the trade name of Rozerem). This works in a somewhat different way from other sleeping tablets, by mimicking the action of melatonin on the brain. Melatonin itself is a hormone which is produced by the brain and plays a role in maintaining the natural cycle of sleeping and waking. Its value in tablet form as a 'natural' sleeping pill has been disputed. It does seem to reduce the length of time it takes a person to get to sleep (although not by very much) but may not be very helpful in ensuring unbroken sleep throughout the night. (See the section on melatonin under the Nutrition Therapy and Supplements heading, later in this book.)

While ramelteon, which mimics melatonin, seems to be relatively safe, it has not yet been shown to be any more effective in humans than melatonin itself, which has the advantage of being much cheaper. Like other sleeping tablets, ramelteon has side effects, including dizziness, headaches and nausea, and it may make symptoms of depression worse.

Antidepressants

Before we go on to look at non-drug therapies, we need to say a word about antidepressants.

The form of insomnia that most frequently occurs in depression is early morning waking – the patient wakes at around 5 am and is unable to get back to sleep again. However, some depressed patients may find difficulty getting to sleep or may be restless during the night. By alleviating the depression, an antidepressant may, of itself, relieve the associated symptoms, such as insomnia. What's more, some antidepressants, such as trazodone (Desyrel, Molipaxin), nefazodone (Serzone), amitriptyline (Elavil, Endep) and mirtazapine (Remeron, Zispin SolTab) have a sedating effect which may help the insomnia even before the antidepressant action kicks in.

Some authorities say that there is little evidence that antidepressants are helpful in the treatment of insomnia unless it is associated with clinical depression. However, because some of them do have a sedating effect, they can also be useful in very small doses in the elderly, since they may be taken safely over a longer period of time than standard hypnotics.

It is usually said that antidepressants are not addictive and do not cause withdrawal effects and, in the case of the tricyclics such as amitriptyline and the MAOIs –

phenelzine sulfate (Nardil), tranylcypromine sulfate (Parnate) and isocarboxazid (Marplan) – which have been around for a very long time, one can be pretty sure that this is so. However, there has been considerable disquiet and a number of court cases concerning paroxetine (Seroxat, Paxil, Asimia), which is one of the newer antidepressants known as SSRI's (selective serotonin reuptake inhibitors). It was originally said to be non-addictive and not to cause withdrawal symptoms but this was subsequently shown to be untrue.

THE ORTHODOX TREATMENT OF OBSTRUCTIVE SLEEP APNEA

If the simple measures suggested in the Do's and Don'ts section don't help, your physician may recommend using continuous positive airway pressure, or CPAP. This consists of a machine which blows a stream of air into the nostrils, via a mask, and so keeps the airways open. Some patients find the masks uncomfortable at first but they are made in different shapes (ranging from a full face mask to one that just fits into the nostrils), sizes and materials, so it should be possible to find one that is comfortable. Some patients like to alternate two different shapes to reduce the risk of them causing irritation. Studies suggest that it is well worth persevering with CPAP if your physician thinks it advisable because it has been shown to improve the quality of sleep, reduce daytime sleepiness, improve the patient's mood and, perhaps most important, reduce the risk of having an automobile accident.

There are various oral appliances available which can be used to move the tongue or the lower jaw in order to open up the airway at the back of the throat. However, these are not universally successful (a recent study showed some improvement in no more than two thirds of patients using them), they can be expensive – and many insurance companies will not pay for them. In addition, depending on where you live, it may be hard to find a dentist who is prepared to fit the appliance and offer the necessary follow-up. For this reason, your physician may not recommend an oral appliance.

If you have a deviated nasal septum or nasal polyps, an operation to correct the first or remove the second may be beneficial.

For patients who have very severe obstructive apnea, an operation may be the most appropriate form of treatment. The simplest of these consists of removal of the uvula (the dangly bit you can see at the back of people's throats if they open their mouths very wide) and part of the soft palate. For patients who have receding chins, an operation that moves the whole jaw forward may be recommended. Although the results of this form of surgery haven't been intensively researched, one study showed that up to 95 per cent of patients who received this treatment had benefited.

Occasionally the obstruction is exacerbated by enlarged tonsils and their removal may greatly improve the condition.

THE ORTHODOX TREATMENT OF RESTLESS LEG SYNDROME AND PERIODIC LIMB MOVEMENTS IN SLEEP

For patients who have symptoms at least three nights a week, drug treatment may be recommended. Some patients have spontaneous remissions which can last weeks or even months and, in these cases, drugs may be prescribed for them to take just when the symptoms are bad.

There is quite a range of drugs that can be used and these fall into six groups – dopaminergic agents, dopamine agonists, benzodiazepines, opioids, anticonvulsants and presynaptic alpha 2 adrenergic agonists. As far as the patient is concerned, the only important thing is that there is more choice within some groups than others and the side effects of the drugs will vary according to which group they fall into.

It's usual to begin with a dopaminergic agent or dopamine agonist and, if these make the symptoms worse (as they can do in some cases) to try benzodiazepines, the anticonvulsant gabapentin or opiates.

Where the condition has arisen as a symptom of kidney failure, it may resolve once the patient has received a transplant.

Dopaminergic agents
Levodopa with carbidopa (Sinemet) can relieve the

symptoms of both PLMS and RLS where there is no underlying cause but can also be helpful for patients who have RLS as a result of kidney disease. The dose is very important because, although up to 200 mg a day is therapeutic, once the dose goes higher than this is will make the symptoms worse in around 85 per cent of patients. There are certain situations in which it is inadvisable to use levodopa (for example in patients with narrow angle glaucoma, melanoma or those taking MAOIs for the treatment of depression). It has not been shown conclusively whether it is safe in pregnancy and it may cause problems in patients with asthma, peptic ulcer or certain heart conditions. Because the absorption of levodopa is affected by the amount of protein in the diet, patients need to try to distribute their protein intake fairly evenly between meals.

Dopamine agonists

These are less likely than levodopa to make the symptoms worse and they can be used with levodopa should this happen. However, they do have side effects of their own, including nausea, light headedness, drowsiness, and dizziness when getting up from lying down. Of course, it's important to remember that not everyone who takes a particular drug will experience the side effects but it's just as well to be aware of them so that you can report them to your physician should they occur.

The dopamine agonists include bromocriptine mesylate (Parlodel), pramipexole (Mirapex), ropinirole hydrochloride (Requip) and pergolide mesylate (Permax). Parlodel tends to produce nausea and dizziness in a lot of patients and so is probably the least useful. Mirapex isn't suitable for patients with kidney failure. Permax is probably the most useful in the treatment of RLS and PLMS, is usually safe to take in pregnancy and can work in patients who haven't responded to levodopa. However, it can cause a variety of side effects from a running nose and indigestion to confusion, palpitations or even hallucinations. For this reason it's unwise for people who are already suffering from confusion to take it

Benzodiazepines

We've already talked about this class of drugs in the section on the drug treatment of insomnia. However, they can also be used to treat RLS and PLMS and, in severe cases, can be combined with another drug. The benzodiazepines most likely to be prescribed are clonazepam (Klonopin), temazepam (Restoril) and alprazolam (Xanax). It seems possible that they work not by actually reducing the symptoms of RLS or PLMS but rather by helping the patient to sleep despite the symptoms.

The same words of warning regarding contraindications, side effects and withdrawal symptoms that have been noted in the section on insomnia treatment are, of course, just as relevant here.

Opioids

Drugs such as codeine or propoxyphene (Darvon, Dolene) can help mild or intermittent symptoms. More powerful preparations such as oxycodone hydrochloride (Roxicodone), methadone hydrochloride (Dolophine) and levorphanol tartrate (Levo-Dromoran) may be used for patients who haven't responded to anything else. However, particularly with the more powerful drugs, great caution is necessary because of the risk of addiction.

Anticonvulsants

These may be helpful when the patient experiences severe muscle spasms. Gabapentin (Neurontin) is useful for patients whose symptoms include pain or other disturbances of sensation (such as tingling or numbness). It can be given on its own or in combination with another drug and is usually well tolerated although it may cause transient sleepiness, dizziness, unsteadiness or fatigue. It is probably best avoided in patients with kidney failure and should not be taken within two hours of antacids which will reduce its absorption.

Presynaptic alpha 2 adrenergic agonists

Clonidine hydrochloride (Catapres) can be effective in RLS where there is no underlying cause and also in cases associated with kidney failure but it has no effect on PLMS. Common side effects include a dry mouth, lightheadedness, sleepiness, constipation and difficulty thinking straight.

ORTHODOX & COMPLEMENTARY TREATMENT OF NIGHT TERRORS & NARCOLEPSY

Night Terrors

It is sensible to try to avoid those facts that may precipitate an episode. So, for children, fevers should be treated promptly, while in adults, alcohol, late nights and large meals eaten late in the evening should be avoided. Sometimes psychotherapy may help. Some doctors recommend Benadryl Elixir for children. In severe cases, in children or adults, an antidepressant or a sedative may be prescribed.

Among the complementary therapies, hypnotherapy, herbal preparations of chamomile or St. John's wort, and aromatherapy have been found to help some patients.

Narcolepsy

The orthodox treatment of narcolepsy consists of stimulants such as amphetamine. However, if the patient can arrange to take regular short naps during the course of the day, the need for such drugs may be reduced. Other symptoms will respond to tricyclic antidepressants, such as imipramine. Lifestyle changes may also play a role and include increasing exercise and reducing stress. Some people find they function better if they work at night and sleep during the day.

Research into narcolepsy is ongoing. It is only recently that evidence has been found for the involvement of hypocretin and it seems likely that future research will now be able to suggest more effective ways of treating the condition.

Complementary therapies that have been found to help some patients include homeopathy, herbalism and acupuncture. Supplements of vitamin B6 have also proved beneficial in some cases.

BEHAVIOR THERAPY

In recent years, when treating patients suffering from insomnia, physicians have increasingly recommended behavior therapy instead of, or in addition to, sleeping tablets. And here we start getting into the realm of self-help treatment because a lot of the things that a behavior therapist will advise you to do, you can try out for yourself right now.

First of all, though, we need to look at what is meant by behavior therapy.

Behavior therapy takes a number of forms: cognitive therapy, relaxation therapy, stimulus control therapy, paradoxical intention therapy and sleep restriction therapy.

These are all used in the treatment of primary insomnia – in other words, when the reason for sleeplessness is not pain or problems with the breathing, or any of the other conditions listed above. This is not to say that it cannot be helpful when the insomnia *is* being caused by something else but it is essential that the "something else" is treated first, and then behavior therapy may help to get you back into the way of sleeping normally.

Cognitive therapy is all about changing your perceptions of yourself and of your sleeping habits. You will be helped to investigate your beliefs about sleep – why you're not sleeping, how much sleep you actually need, what time you should go to bed and so on – and to see which of these beliefs are helping to perpetuate the problem. Having gained this insight, you will then be helped to introduce healthier beliefs and behavior patterns into your life.

Relaxation therapy is exactly what it says it is. You are taught how to deal with the tensions that are keeping you awake. There are a number of methods including progressive muscle relaxation, biofeedback techniques, breathing techniques, visualization techniques and meditation. (Meditation will be covered further in the section on complementary medicine.)

Progressive muscle relaxation is simply a system of first tensing and then relaxing groups of muscles, progressing through the body. The initial tensing is important because it helps you to appreciate the difference between a fully tensed muscle and a relaxed (or semi-relaxed) one.

Biofeedback techniques use machinery to show you visually how effective your efforts to relax are. You will be linked to a monitor that records blood pressure, heart rate and other variables and, as you find the right way in which to relax, the monitor will show a drop in blood pressure or a reduction in muscle tension. After some practice, you will be able to identify exactly what is necessary in order to bring about the desired effect.

Breathing techniques teach you to copy the slow shallow breathing that occurs with the onset of sleep. Some meditation techniques also involve the breath and these will be covered later on.

Stimulus control therapy is about reassociating the bedroom and bed with the idea of sleepiness in your unconscious mind. We've already covered one of the problems associated with insomnia – the dread of going to bed and having yet another sleepless night. In this state of mind, you are anything but sleepy when you go to bed and the chances are that you'll sit in bed reading or watching television in the hope of "drifting off", which just makes matters worse by stimulating your mind still further.

The first rule of stimulus control therapy is: Don't use the bedroom for anything other than sleeping and sex. Now, it might be thought that sex was far more likely to arouse you than to calm you. However, the arousal that occurs while you're actually having sex is quickly replaced by a very relaxed state once you've finished (hence all the old jokes about men just turning over and going to sleep straight away). But television and reading and drinking cups of tea stimulate rather than relax, so they need to be banned from the bedroom.

The second rule is: Go to bed only when you're sleepy and then, if you haven't fallen asleep within 20 to 30 minutes, get up again and do something relaxing (such as listening to soft music) until you feel sleepy again. It's important during this time to avoid bright light, so if you don't have a dimmer switch, just put on a table light with a low wattage bulb. Then once you're sleepy again, return to bed. But if you still can't sleep, repeat the procedure – and keep on doing it until, eventually, you do fall asleep.

It's also important that you don't spend more time in bed than necessary – if you lie awake in bed, your subconscious will continue to associate being in bed with the idea of sleeplessness. It's also important to get up at the same time each day, no matter how little sleep you've had. And if you possibly can, avoid daytime naps. This may all sound a bit stressful but clinical trials have shown that stimulus control therapy can be very effective both for patients who have difficulty falling asleep and for those who have long sleepless periods during the night.

Paradoxical intention therapy alleviates anxiety by getting you willingly to experience whatever it is that you most fear – in the case of insomnia, this means staying awake all night. However, this is a technique that needs to be done under the guidance of a qualified therapist.

Sleep restriction therapy is what it says it is. You may think that, if you suffer from insomnia, the last thing you want is to have what little sleep you do get curtailed. However, this therapy, like stimulus control therapy, is all about retraining the unconscious mind in order to allow sleeping patterns to improve. As we noted above, lying in bed wide awake for prolonged periods can make insomnia worse.

First of all you will be asked to try to assess accurately the actual length of time you spend asleep each night. You will then be told that you must stay in bed no longer than that – if you sleep only five hours then, if you go to bed at midnight, you must get up at five in the morning, whether you've slept or not. This is likely to make you feel very tired the following day with the result that, when you go to bed the following night, you'll fall asleep more readily. As your sleeping patterns improve, you will be allowed to spend longer in bed, the amount being increased gradually by 15 to 30 minutes at a time. This is done over a period of several weeks and normally it is the bedtime that is changed and the getting up time which remains the same.

Self-help: If you want to try behavior therapy techniques for yourself, the best one to use is stimulus control therapy. The others will probably achieve better results if used under the supervision of a therapist and some, such as cognitive therapy, cannot be done as self-help programs.

ORTHODOX TREATMENT OF CIRCADIAN RHYTHM DISORDERS

Because these disorders are rare, I am only including advice about orthodox treatment. This is not to say that complementary therapies would not be helpful. If you wanted to go down this route, homoeopathy or acupuncture would probably be worth trying. However, the rarity of the conditions mean that I am unable to say exactly what, within these therapies, would be likely to help.

Delayed Sleep Phase Disorder (DSPD)

There are several ways in which DSPD can be treated. The patient is allowed to sleep until he wakes spontaneously and, as soon as he is awake, sits in a strong light for between 30 and 90 minutes. Although this is effective, it has to be continued indefinitely. However, some people are able, after a while, to make do with just 15 minutes a day or may only have to use the light a few times a week, or even just a few times a month. In the evening, the light needs to be dimmed and this is reinforced by the patient wearing amber-coloured glasses which prevent blue light from reaching the eyes.

Melatonin is often prescribed in small doses taken an hour or so before bedtime. Recently, a sleeping tablet has been developed called ramelteon (Rozerem) which acts in a similar way to melatonin and may therefore be helpful.

A third method of treatment is 'sleep phase chronotherapy' which consists of changing the patient's bedtime over a series of nights until the desired time is reached. However, this has to be repeated at regular intervals and the long term effects are unclear.

Advanced Sleep Phase Disorder (ASPD)

The primary treatment for ASPD consists of bright light therapy in the early evening, at the time when the patient usually starts to feel sleepy. The light is then withdrawn later in the evening, allowing normal sleepiness to develop.

Irregular Sleep Wake Rhythm

Various treatments have been used for this problem, including melatonin, increased light during the daytime, and maintaining a regular timetable of activities throughout the day.

Non 24 Hour Sleep Wake Disorder (N24HSWD) or Hypernychtemeral Syndrome

For the few sighted people who suffer from this disorder, light treatment can be helpful. Melatonin is useful for both sighted and blind people and needs to be given at exactly the same time every night. Studies have shown that a dose of 0.5 mg given at a set time between 6pm and 9pm are most effective. However, this is not something that should be tried as a self-help treatment. In order to achieve the best results, melatonin needs to be of a pharmaceutical grade (to ensure which, it should be prescribed) and should be administered under the supervision of a sleep specialist.

A major breakthrough has been the licencing of the drug tasimelteon (Hetlioz) which has a melatonin-like action and was approved by the FDA, solely for the treatment of N24HSWD in blind people, in January 2014.

END OF PART THREE

PART FOUR – WHAT ELSE CAN HELP? USING COMPLEMENTARY MEDICINE

 Many forms of complementary medicine can be used as self-help therapies. And since most of them are free of side effects, they are perfectly safe to use. However, if you have any suspicion that your insomnia is due to an underlying medical or psychological cause, you should speak to your physician before trying any form of therapy. Once you've been checked out, it's then up to you to decide what treatment you want to use but, as I've already mentioned, you do need to understand your own insomnia in order to make the best decision as to treatment.

ACUPUNCTURE

A brief introduction

When you're looking for a treatment for insomnia, acupuncture is unlikely to be the first thing that springs to mind. Most people have heard that it's an effective treatment for pain but many are unaware that it has a much wider scope than that. However, it has long been known as a useful treatment for insomnia, especially in the elderly. Some reports have suggested that the success rate is nearly 90 per cent and that, in the case of the elderly, not only do they wake up less often during the night but their quality of sleep improves.

Acupuncture was developed in China over two thousand years ago and was first brought to the West in the seventeenth century by merchants who traveled to the East under the auspices of the great trading companies. However, although a number of doctors in France, Italy, Germany and elsewhere became interested in acupuncture and some even wrote books on the subject, the therapy was not widely practiced in Europe during this period.

In the nineteenth century acupuncture was again brought to the West by Chinese immigrants, but as they only used it within their own communities, there was no resurgence of interest. However, in 1972 when President Nixon was shown acupuncture in action during the course of his visit to China, the therapy finally caught the imagination of, first, the media and then the general public in the West. Nowadays there are many established acupuncture training colleges and qualified acupuncturists throughout the West.

The idea behind acupuncture is one of energy balance. The vital force (the energy whose presence or absence makes the difference between a living person and a dead body) is known in Chinese as Qi (pronounced "chee") and is said to run through the body in a system of channels or meridians. There are twelve pairs of major meridians, each named after the organ with which they are connected (such as the Lung meridian and the Liver meridian) and two meridians which run along the midline of the body, back and front, meeting to form a circle.

When the flow of energy in these meridians becomes disrupted, disease results. Painful conditions are frequently due to a blockage in the flow. But Qi can be affected in other ways as well – there can be a deficiency or an excess in one or more meridians or there can be an imbalance of yin and yang.

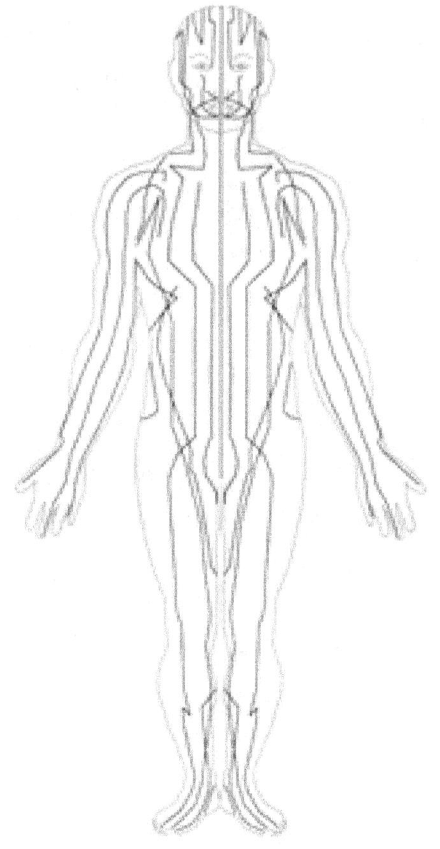

Diagram showing the approximate course of the acupuncture meridians on the front of the front of the body

Yin and yang are not things in themselves but aspects of everything – rather like left and right or up and down. And for good health, it is essential that the yin and yang of the body and of Qi be in perfect balance. Thinking of it in terms of right and left, if the three shapes below were solid blocks, the only one which was stable and not in imminent danger of toppling over, would be the one in the center. The shape on the left has too much "right" and the shape on the right has too much "left".

There is a third way in which Qi can be disrupted and this is by being affected by external factors (sometimes known as harmful Qi). There are six external factors – wind, cold, damp, dryness, heat and damp heat. Skeptics sometimes point to these concepts as proving that acupuncture is "non-scientific" but, although centuries ago people no doubt believed that the body was, in fact, being invaded by these factors, nowadays they are used simply as a shorthand to describe what is happening to the body and to indicate what treatment is necessary. For example, someone with a raging fever has been affected by heat, and someone with a streaming cold and a heavy feeling in the head has been affected by damp. Invasion by wind, however, produces symptoms that have the characteristics of wind, constantly changing and moving, and doesn't necessarily cause flatulence!

The acupuncturist will look at the patient's tongue and feel the pulse in order to confirm the diagnosis. This is a far more complicated affair than in Western medicine. Whereas the

Western physician is simply looking at the tongue to ensure that it is moist (and the patient isn't dehydrated) and pink (and not blue which would indicate inadequate oxygen in the bloodstream), the acupuncturist looks at the color, the coating and the physical appearance of the tongue.

And whereas the Western physician feels the pulse with two fingers to assess the rate and the rhythm, the acupuncturist will use three fingers spaced apart to determine the characteristics of six pulses in each wrist (each reflecting the condition of Qi in one of the twelve major meridians). And he will not be feeling just for rate and rhythm but for one of 30 or more different qualities of pulse – such as superficial or deep, rough or slippery, wiry, knotted or moving. By checking each of the twelve pulses against each other the acupuncturist can assess not only the health of the individual meridians but their relationship to each other in terms of Qi and also the quality of Qi in the organs of the body. Little wonder that it takes years of training to become a proficient acupuncturist!

The acupuncturist's view of insomnia

According to acupuncture theory, when we go to bed, it is normal for blood (or fluid) to move from the yang system into the yin system. (Yin is associated with the inside, darkness, quietness, cold and night-time, yang with the outside, brightness, activity, heat and daytime.) In the morning, blood flows back out to the external body surface and we wake up. The idea of yin being dominant at night is reflected in the fact that being too hot or too active (mentally or physically) will keep you awake.

The major organs that relate to blood in the Chinese system are the Spleen, Heart and Liver. (These are given capital letters because they relate as much to the energy of these organs as to the physical organs themselves.) But one of these – the Heart – controls the emotions so that emotional problems, stress or overwork can interfere with the normal flow of blood. As a result, the blood doesn't flow into yin at night and sleep is disrupted.

Acupuncture treatment for insomnia

Because acupuncture is a holistic therapy which takes account of the whole patient, any treatment will be tailor-made for that particular patient. It is impossible, therefore, to give a list of treatments (as can be done with, say, sleeping pills) and say that one of these will be used for a patient complaining of insomnia. However, there are certain combinations of symptoms which may often be found in insomnia:

- Sleep which is disturbed by dreams, headaches, discomfort in the upper part of the abdomen, a bitter taste in the mouth, and a tendency to get upset or angry very easily are all symptoms of stagnation in the Liver which results in Heat that attacks the Heart (or mind). The diagnosis would be confirmed if the acupuncturist found that your tongue was red with a yellow coating and that your pulse was wiry and rapid. The treatment is to expel the Heat, soothe the Liver and calm the mind.

- If you tend to be irritable and, as well as insomnia, you suffer from dizziness and low back pain and have a rapid, weak pulse, a diagnosis may be made of disharmony of the Heart and Kidney. Treatment aims to restore harmony.

- When, as well as insomnia, you have a feeling of fullness or bloating and belching and you also have a history of eating an irregular diet, and if, on examination, the acupuncturist finds a slippery rapid pulse and a red tongue with a yellow greasy coat, the diagnosis is likely to be that of Phlegm and Heat attacking the Heart. The treatment is to expel the Phlegm and Heat and calm the mind.

- Light sleep, disturbing dreams, palpitations, poor memory, listlessness and a poor appetite are all symptoms of a deficiency of Qi and of Blood in the Heart and Spleen. The tongue is pale with a thin coating and the pulse is thin and weak. Here it is necessary to nourish the Qi and the Blood and to calm the heart.

The combination of needles used in any one case will depend on the type of insomnia which has been diagnosed. However, there are two points which will be used in many cases. These are the seventh point on the Heart meridian (known as H 7 and also called the "Door of the mind") which lies on the wrist, and the sixth point along the Spleen meridian (Sp 6) which is situated on the inside of the leg just above the ankle. The first of these points calms the mind while the second stimulates yin which, as was mentioned above, needs to be dominant at night if you're to get a good night's sleep.

In addition to these two, other points will be used according to the diagnosis:

- A point on the Liver meridian, Liver 2 (usually abbreviated to Liv 2), which lies between the first and second toes can be used to reduce Heat and clear stagnation.

- Stagnation can also be cleared by two points on the Bladder meridian (Bl 18 and Bl 19), which are situated on the back a little way above the waist.

- Two other Bladder points, Bl 15 and Bl 23 used together will balance the Qi between the Heart and Kidney. Both are on the back, lying along a line that runs parallel to the spinal column, one at around waist level and the other a little higher than armpit level.

- Bl 15 can also be used to strengthen the Qi of the Heart when there is a deficiency, while Bl 20, lying on the same line parallel to the spinal column and a little above the waist, will stimulate the Spleen and promote the circulation of Qi.

- To dispel Phlegm, a point on the Stomach meridian (St

40), on the side of the leg immediately below the calf, may be used.

The acupuncturist will choose the combination of points that seem to offer the most appropriate treatment for the individual patient. This may include other points on the arms, legs or trunk in addition to, or instead of, those mentioned above. Every patient is different and so every patient will be treated differently. However, it is unusual for more than six or eight needles to be used at any one time.

Ear acupuncture

As an alternative to standard acupuncture, ear acupuncture can be used to treat insomnia. The system of ear acupuncture, or auriculotherapy, was developed in the mid 20th century by Dr. Thomas Nogier, a Frenchman. The idea behind it is that the whole body is reflected in microcosm in the ear (this is similar to the theory of reflexology which sees the body reflected in the hands and feet). So a single needle in the ear may be used to treat a localized or specific condition. This can be particularly useful when treating young children or other patients who aren't over-fond of needles, although it's most effective when used in combination with standard acupuncture treatments.

Ear acupuncture can be used to help weight loss and to aid people to stop smoking, as well as being useful in the treatment of insomnia. In all three cases, a small stud which resembles a tiny thumb-tack is inserted into the relevant point on the ear and left there, held in by a piece of sticky tape.

There is a particular point in the ear called Shenmen which is used for the treatment of insomnia. About an hour before going to bed, the patient massages the stud and thus stimulates the point. The great advantage of using an ear stud is that it can be used as often as necessary so, if you wake in the night, you can massage it again to send yourself back to sleep.

Self-help techniques using acupuncture points

It may seem a little strange to have a paragraph on self-help in the section on acupuncture. After all, you can't stick needles in yourself very easily and, anyway, it takes several years of training to learn the position of the points and which to use in which circumstances.

However, there is a technique known as acupressure in which the points are stimulated not by needles but by massage. And since, as we have seen, there are two points which are commonly used for the treatment of all types of insomnia, no harm can come from a little self-administered massage of these points. The massage should be of the type known as "pulsed pressure" – you press firmly on the point for a few seconds, then let go, then press again, and continue pressing and letting go for about two minutes. The points may be tender at first – points that need treating are often painful. The Chinese call them "Ah-shi" points (meaning "oh, yes!!"). The English version used by some acupuncturists is "ouch" points.

To find Heart 7 hold one of your hands (it doesn't matter which) face up. You will see a crease running across your wrist. (There may be several creases, but this is the most obvious one, nearest to the palm.) Gently run the thumb of your other hand along this crease starting at the side nearest your little finger. Almost immediately you will feel a ridge formed by a tendon. (This becomes even more obvious if you bend your hand up.) Once your thumb has slid over this tendon, it is over H7 (roughly in a line with your third finger).

To find Sp 6, with your palm facing downwards, grasp your opposite leg, so that the V between your thumb and first finger is around the back of your ankle. Adjust your hand so that your fingers are lying horizontally and the lower border of your little finger is level with the middle of the bulge made by the ankle bone. Sp 6 lies at the level of upper border of your index finger, in line with the ankle bone.

When you use pulsed pressure, it is important not to overdo it. Two minutes on one wrist and two minutes on one leg should be enough to begin with. If you find it helpful, you can experiment to see whether using it for slightly longer or slightly less produces better effects. If it hasn't worked after five or six days, stop using it.

Even if pulsed pressure hasn't helped, this doesn't mean that acupuncture itself won't be effective. But, if it helps partially, then acupuncture is probably the treatment of choice to effect a complete cure.

[For a fuller description of acupuncture, its history and the ways in which it can treat a wide variety of diseases, see my book *Is Acupuncture Right For You?*, published by Inner Traditions.]

AROMATHERAPY

Aromatherapy involves the use of scented oils and, while not having the capacity to treat such a wide variety of ailments as some other therapies, it can be very useful in conditions associated with tension or anxiety. You can try treating yourself or, if your insomnia is severe, you might find it better to consult an aromatherapist.

The oils can be used:

- as an **inhalation**: put between six and ten drops of the oil into a bowl of steaming water, bend over the bowl with a towel over your head (to keep the steam in), close your eyes (to prevent the oil from irritating them) and inhale for about five minutes.

- as a **diffusion**: you can buy a diffuser, which consists of a small container that fits over a candle. Fill the container with water and add six to ten drops of oil, then light the candle.

- as an **air freshener**: put two fluid ounces of water into a spray bottle, add around 50 drops of oil and shake well before spraying into the air.

- in a **bath**: put eight to ten drops of oil into a tub of water and stir it round before getting in. Because the oil may react with soap, use this bath just to relax in rather than to wash.

- for a **massage**: mix five to ten drops of oil with five teaspoons of a light unscented oil such as cold pressed sunflower oil or sweet almond oil. Or mix three drops of oil with a couple of teaspoons of unscented body lotion. It's advisable not to use either of these on your face unless recommended by an aromatherapist. And always make sure that the mixture is thoroughly blended before you use it because a strong concentration of aromatherapy oils can irritate the skin. If you are giving a child a massage, you should use only half the number of drops suggested.

- on a **tissue**: put one or two drops on a tissue and put it next to your pillow. (Don't put it on your pillow as contact with your face might cause irritation.)

There is quite a variety of oils that can be used to treat insomnia:

- **benzoin** has a sedative effect and will make you feel warm and relaxed. It is particularly useful for treating insomnia which is due to worry, tension or emotional exhaustion. However, some people are sensitive to the oil so use it cautiously to begin with.

- **bergamot** is used to treat anxiety, depression, grief, itchy skin, symptoms of both PMS and the menopause, and stress. It refreshes and relaxes but needs to be used with caution because skin which has been treated with bergamot oil may become sensitive to sunlight.

- **chamomile.** Most people know that chamomile (or camomile – both spellings are used) is a relaxant when made into a tea. The oil has similar effects. Because it is also useful in the treatment of stress, anxiety and tension, arthritic and muscular pain, backache, depression, grief, headaches and migraine, menopausal hot flashes, indigestion, irritability, itchy skin and jet lag, it can be used to treat insomnia which is due to any of these causes. Like benzoin, it can cause dermatitis (irritated skin) in some people, so use with caution to begin with. Chamomile should not be used during the first few months of pregnancy.

- **clary sage** is used for anxiety, backache and other muscular aches and pains, depression, exhaustion, headaches and migraine, menopausal symptoms, muscle spasm, stress and tension. Clary sage may also improve the memory. It shouldn't be used during pregnancy or by anyone who has a condition known to be affected by estrogen (for example, some types of cancer). If you are taking estrogen in the form of HRT or the contraceptive pill, ask the advice of a qualified aromatherapist before using clary sage.

- **geranium** lifts the mood and relaxes. It's used for anxiety, depression, exhaustion, grief, muscular aches and pains, stress or tension, and insomnia associated with any of these.

- **jasmine** can be helpful in depression and exhaustion, and is also used to treat apathy, grief, stress, tension, catarrh, muscular aches and pains, and breathing difficulties, and for insomnia associated with any of these conditions.

- **lavender** is used to treat arthritic and muscular pain, backache, depression, exhaustion, fatigue, headaches and migraine, menopausal hot flashes, catarrh, irritability, itchy skin, restlessness, stress, tension, shock, anxiety and jet lag. It has a powerful calming effect and soothes both the nervous system and the digestion as well as being able to relieve pain and lower a raised blood pressure. Not only can it improve the quality of sleep, but it can also result in a more stable mood and an ability to think more clearly. A study which compared patients who received a massage with lavender to another group who just received the massage found that those who had the lavender felt less anxious and more positive after treatment than those in the other group.

- **lemon** is used for arthritic pain, depression, lack of energy, exhaustion, headaches and migraine, menopausal symptoms, stress and tension. It lifts the mood, soothes and refreshes. However, it may irritate sensitive skin or, like bergamot, make the skin sensitive to sunlight, so use it cautiously to begin with.

- **lemon balm** or **melissa** is relaxing and uplifting. It can lower raised blood pressure, aid the digestion and help in the treatment of anxiety, coughs, depression, nervous tension, shock, and even an overactive thyroid. It can cause skin irritation so use it cautiously to begin with.

- **neroli** can be used for insomnia due to anxiety, depression, irritability, panic or shock.

- **orange** is used to treat anxiety, depression, lack of energy and exhaustion, indigestion, muscular aches and pains, nervousness, stress or tension, and insomnia due to any of these causes.

- **rose** is relaxing and soothing as anyone who has sat for any time in a garden full of scented roses will know. The oil is used for insomnia, anxiety, tension, depression, headaches and migraine, muscular aches and pains, stress and asthma.

- **sandalwood** has an antidepressant effect and soothes the digestive and nervous systems. It's used to treat anxiety, depression, indigestion, menopausal symptoms, stress, tension and catarrh, as well as insomnia.

- **sweet marjoram** has a warming and comforting effect. It aids the digestion and is used to treat insomnia, anxiety, headaches, catarrh and pain in the muscles and joints.

- **tangerine** is for anxiety, depression, indigestion, muscular aches and pains, stress and nervousness. It refreshes and relaxes but may cause the skin to become sensitive to sunlight, so use it cautiously.

- **ylang ylang** has the ability to lift the patient's mood and to relax and soothe. It's antidepressant and it can help to lower a raised blood pressure. It's used to treat anxiety, depression, exhaustion, fatigue, irritability, menopausal problems, muscular aches and pains, stress, tension, restlessness and insomnia due to any of these conditions.

If there are medical or psychological reasons for your insomnia (and you have already talked to your physician about it) you can use the chart on the next page to decide which oil is most appropriate for you. **The aromas which are in lower case italics (eg ben) are those which may cause sensitivity or which should not be used in certain cases, as stated in the section above.**

However, if you feel that yours is a simple insomnia, not being caused by any underlying conditions, you may find that simply using four or five drops each of two of the relaxing oils, such as chamomile and rose or chamomile and geranium, in a bath an hour or two before bedtime may be very helpful.

	Worry, tension, *stress*, anxiety	Depression, grief	Itchy skin	Menopause, PMS	Arthritis, muscular aches & pains	Headache, migraine
ben	✓					
ber	✓	✓	✓	✓		
ch	✓	✓	✓	✓	✓	✓
cs	✓	✓		✓	✓	✓
GER	✓	✓			✓	
JAS	✓	✓			✓	
LAVE	✓	✓	✓	✓	✓	✓
lem	✓	✓		✓	✓	✓
lb	✓	✓				
NER	✓	✓				
ORA	✓	✓			✓	
ROS	✓	✓			✓	✓
SAN	✓	✓		✓		
SM	✓				✓	✓
tan	✓	✓			✓	
YY	✓	✓		✓	✓	

Summary of specific uses of aromatherapy oils

AYURVEDIC MEDICINE

A brief introduction

Ayurvedic medicine is the traditional system used in India. It has become increasingly popular in the West in recent years thanks to advocates such as Dr. Deepak Chopra, an endocrinologist who played a large part in introducing Ayurveda into the United States.

According to the basic theory of Ayurveda, all living organisms are regulated by three biological forces – Vata, Pitta and Kapha – which are known collectively as the doshas. Everyone is made up of Vata, Pitta and Kapha but while, in a truly healthy body, all three forces will be in balance, in most people one dosha is dominant. Imbalance, which can be due either to an excess or a deficiency, is the cause of disease.

Each dosha is said to be composed of two elements – Vata is space and air, Pitta is fire and water, and Kapha is water and earth, and it is from these elements that they acquire their individual qualities.

Vata dosha, composed of space and air, is light and subtle and moving. It channels sight through the eyes and sound through the ears and is responsible for sensations. It also governs everything that moves within the body, such as the movement of air in and out of the lungs, the circulation of blood around the body, the movement of food through the digestive system, and the constant flow of thoughts through the mind. Symptoms of excess Vata include:

- digestive disturbances resulting from abnormal movement (so flatulence or constipation)

- cough, shortness of breath

- lack of energy, apathy, fatigue

- dulling of the senses

- anxiety, poor memory, restlessness, inability to relax or to concentrate

- insomnia

Pitta dosha, composed of fire and water, is responsible for what Western physicians would call the metabolic processes, as well as governing the intellect, will power and our ability to perceive reality. Symptoms of excess Pitta include:

- digestive problems resulting from abnormal metabolism (so peptic ulcer, irritable bowel syndrome, diarrhea)

- poor vision

- unhealthy or yellow skin

- disturbed body temperature, excessive sweating

- lack of energy, apathy

- irritability, anxiety, obsession

- dullness of the mind

- irresponsibility, lack of discipline

The third dosha, Kapha, which is made up of water and earth provides structure and is responsible for the strength, stability and endurance of both the body and the mind.

It controls the body's ability to cope with illness, being responsible not only for the immune system but also for the body's ability to heal itself. And it also acts to prevent the other two doshas, Vata and Pitta, from becoming excessive. Symptoms of excessive Kapha include:

- dryness of the mouth and skin

- poor physique

- obesity

- reduced resistance to infections

- tendency to sprained joints

- intolerance, rudeness, jealousy, insecurity

Although I have briefly outlined all three doshas here, in order to give some idea of the theory of Ayurvedic medicine, you will have noticed that only one excessive state – that of Vata – causes insomnia. And because sleeplessness has the effect of increasing Vata, insomnia can – as we have already observed – become a vicious cycle.

Ayurvedic treatment

In treating insomnia, the Ayurvedic physician will use a two-pronged attack which consists of prescribing herbal remedies and recommending changes to diet and lifestyle, all of which will reduce Vata.

One of the herbs most commonly used is Brahmi (Bacopa Monniera) which is a succulent creeper that grows throughout India. It is used primarily to treat nervous tension and insomnia and is also said to clear the mind and enhance learning and concentration.

Another herb, which is sometimes used together with Brahmi, is Shankhpushpi (also spelled Shankapushpi) which has been used in India for centuries to treat anxiety, stress and insomnia.

Although such herbs are widely available over the counter and on the Internet, it is advisable, if you want to try Ayurvedic herbal treatment, to consult a qualified practitioner. In this way you will ensure that you receive the herbs and dosages that are right for you personally. However, the lifestyle and dietary changes can be used as a self-help treatment.

Ayurvedic self-help treatment

Vata can be thrown out of balance by excessive exercise or excessive sexual activity, by fasting or not eating enough, and by staying up late. The first requirement, therefore, is to try to achieve moderation in all things. In addition, a regular daily routine will help to keep Vata in balance. Daily meditation may help to calm the mind. (Meditation methods are covered in a separate section later on.)

Just before bedtime, massage some warm oil (such as sesame or jasmine) into your scalp and the soles of your feet for a few minutes. And drink some warm milk flavored with a pinch of nutmeg, a pinch of cardamom and some crushed almonds.

According to Ayurvedic theory, the 24 hour daily cycle is divided into six periods, during each of which one of the doshas is dominant. The easiest period in which to fall asleep is that of Kapha which has a natural quality of heaviness. Because Kapha rules the hours between 6.00 and 10.00 (both am and pm), this suggests that going to bed before 10 o'clock will give a greater chance of falling asleep easily. After 10.00 the cycle moves into Pitta whose qualities of liveliness and mental alertness are not conducive to falling asleep. Most of us can remember times when we have felt quite drowsy early in the evening, only to wake up later on.

Because an early bedtime is recommended, supper should be eaten early and the main meal should be taken at midday.

You might reasonably feel that a regime of light suppers and early nights is not something that you would want to continue for the rest of your life. But if you can follow it for a period of weeks until you are sleeping better, then the occasional late night can be introduced. Eventually, once you are sleeping well on a regular basis, you can start to get back to a regime that is more conducive to your way of life. However, you should continue to do as much as possible to keep Vata in balance so that the insomnia doesn't recur.

One of the main ways in which you can do this is to eat a "Vata-pacifying" diet. This consists mainly of warm food with moderately heavy textures, together with milk, cream and butter. Eat a good breakfast and, in the late afternoon, have a cup of herbal tea with a snack. The foods that are good to eat are:

- soups

- stews and casseroles

- fresh bread

- sweet fruits

- cooked vegetables apart from those listed below under "foods that should be avoided"

- oats, rice, wheat

- chicken, turkey, tofu, seafood

- chickpeas, mung beans, pink lentils

- nuts and seeds

The foods that should be avoided are:

- cold foods

- raw vegetables

- candy

* unripe fruit

* cabbage and brussels sprouts

* broccoli, cauliflower, celery, eggplant, leafy green vegetables, mushrooms, peas, peppers, potatoes, sprouts, tomatoes and zucchini unless they have been cooked with a little oil

* apples, cranberries and pears unless cooked

* dried fruit

* barley, buckwheat, corn (maize), millet, rye

* red meat

* bitter or astringent herbs such as coriander seed, fenugreek, parsley, saffron and turmeric

BACH & OTHER FLOWER REMEDIES

Flower remedies cannot be said to offer specific treatment for insomnia, but for some of the conditions that can cause insomnia – such as anxiety, grief and stress – they can be remarkably effective. One word of caution, though. Most essences use alcohol as a preservative although it is now possible to get some of them in an alcohol-free form. The actual amount of alcohol contained in two drops of remedy is very small but anyone who is very sensitive to alcohol should consult a physician before taking any of the remedies. Alternatively, the remedy can be rubbed into the skin rather than being taken orally.

The Bach remedies are probably the best known of the flower remedies. They were developed in the 1930s by Dr. Edward Bach, a highly qualified and well respected British physician who felt intuitively that some of his patients would get better more quickly if they were in a better frame of mind. His belief that nature could perhaps produce something more than the orthodox medicine of the day had to offer led him to develop 38 flower remedies which are made either by floating the flowers in spring water in strong sunlight or by boiling them in water for a short period. Each remedy is specific for a particular emotional state – for example, White Chestnut will help someone whose mind is constantly going round and round, dwelling on problems, while Mimulus is for fear and anxiety.

Remedies are still produced according to Dr. Bach's methods at the Bach Centre in Oxfordshire, England. If you go to the Centre's website on:
http://www.bachcentre.com/centre/remedies.htm
you will find a list of all the remedies and their uses.

Since Dr. Bach's time, many other people around the world have started to make flower remedies or essences, using similar methods but different flowers. Most of these are now available on the Internet and, if you type "flower essences" into a search engine you will be presented with thousands of websites offering these for sale. If you feel that there's a particular aspect of your emotional state which is contributing to your problems, then it might be worth browsing some of these to find an appropriate remedy. Available remedies include:

- **Red Suva Frangipani** – an *Australian bush flower essence* which is for grief, sadness, emotional upheaval and turmoil particularly when caused by a relationship going sour or the death of a loved one.

- **Cassandra** – an *Alaskan flower essence* which is calming and encourages stillness of mind and is particularly useful for people who are constantly anxious and who find it hard to relax their minds.

- **Lettuce** – one of the *"Spirit-in-Nature"* essences which calms people who are caught up in emotions and which is particularly helpful for those who are highly creative.

- **Grape hyacinth** – a *Pacific essence* which is useful for shock, despair and stress.

- **Gold Waitsia** – found in the *"Living essences of Australia"* range which can alleviate anxiety caused by too much attention to detail and produce a more spontaneous attitude to life. It's also helpful for people who are recovering from illness and are finding it hard to accept their incapacity.

- **Blue Vervain** and **Lavender** – from the *Tree Frog Farm flower essences* range. The effect of the first is described as "let your bitter thoughts rest peacefully while you go floating on the breeze of sweet calm" and that of the second as "sweet dreams are made of these: how you perceive and move through the landscape of your thoughts. Step away and relax into watching the process."

Although there are many complementary practitioners who prescribe flower essences, they are an ideal self-help remedy for the simple reason that they seem to have no side effects whatsoever and can be taken as often as you need them. At the end of a tiring day's work, I find that two drops of Dr. Bach's Olive remedy in a hot drink (Olive being indicated for physical and mental exhaustion) is a remarkably good pick-me-up.

Very occasionally deep rooted emotional problems may come to the surface as a result of taking a flower remedy, or a skin rash may appear. These are both part of the healing process and are indications that the remedy is working. In the vast majority of cases, however, the remedy will just cause a gradual increase in well-being. If it doesn't, this suggests that it's not the right remedy for you, and you should look again.

CHIROPRACTIC

According to chiropractors, the key to a healthy body is a healthy spine and a healthy nervous system. Because the spine carries within it the spinal cord from which nerves are sent out to all areas of the body, problems arising in the spine can cause irritation of the nerves which, in turn, can cause pain and malfunction in other parts of the body. By manipulating the joints and, in particular, those of the spinal column, chiropractors aim to restore the bodily systems to a state of harmony in which the body can heal itself.

Through massage and manipulation, the chiropractor can relieve muscle spasm and other painful conditions that may be contributing to a patient's insomnia. The treatment may also improve the mobility of the chest wall so that breathing becomes easier and more oxygen enters the blood stream, making the patient less restless.

Some chiropractors offer additional therapies in combination with chiropractic, such as herbalism or acupuncture. Acupuncture and chiropractic used together have a very good record of success in the treatment of insomnia.

COLOR THERAPY

Color can have remarkable effects on our state of mind. An experiment done some years ago directed people who had appointments to see a doctor into one of two waiting rooms – one was painted blue, the other yellow. When they were kept waiting beyond their appointment time, the people in the blue room became far less agitated than those in the yellow room.

Think, too, about the colors that have specific associations – dark colors for mourning and as a sign of authority (lawyers, priests, cops, prison staff), red for jollity (Santa Claus), white for purity & cleanliness (wedding dresses, doctors' coats) and you will begin to see what a major role color plays in our lives.

Color therapists tell us that not only do colors affect us emotionally but that they can have a definite therapeutic effect. Some can calm, others can excite (do you think you would sleep better in a room painted a soft blue or one with red and orange stripes?).

You can, of course, use a form of color therapy as a self-help treatment. However, if you see a therapist, a full case history will be taken and a diagnosis made before treatment is given in the form of colored lights shone onto specific parts of your body.

The two colors which are most likely to be used in the treatment of insomnia are blue and violet. The first is relaxing and calming and can actually slow the pulse and reduce high blood pressure. Violet, too, is relaxing and soothing and, in addition, can suppress the appetite. Blue can be used to treat neuralgia and both blue and violet are useful in the treatment of nervous tension, irritability and anxiety.

Although light therapy should always be done under the guidance of a qualified practitioner, making sure that your bedroom is painted in restful colors may also help. Because light is a form of energy, therapists sometimes recommend that patients "energize" drinking water by putting it in a colored glass container and allowing sunlight to shine through it for an hour or so. Since blue glass is relatively easy to acquire, this may be an appropriate way to self-treat using color therapy.

Color can also be used in meditation (of which more is said in a later section). Once you're in bed, close your eyes and visualise yourself surrounded by blue . . . you may like to float in a soft blue cloud or swim in a clear blue lake or stand under a gentle blue waterfall. Just let your imagination take you into the "blueness" and feel it soothing and relaxing you.

CRANIOSACRAL THERAPY (CRANIAL OSTEOPATHY)

A relative newcomer in the world of complementary therapies, craniosacral therapy consists of very gentle manipulation of the bones of the skull. In fact, the manipulation is so gentle that it's often recommended for small children, pregnant women and for the elderly where other manipulative therapies may be inappropriate.

Originally called cranial osteopathy because of the focus on the skull, or cranium, the newer title – craniosacral therapy – reflects the development of the treatment to include the pelvis and the spine. The therapist locates areas of strain and imbalance and uses the gentlest of pressure to release and rebalance them. Such strains and tensions may be the cause not only of physical conditions such as back pain, migraine or digestive problems but also anxiety or depression.

Many of the conditions that respond well to craniosacral therapy – such as arthritis, asthma and other breathing problems, back pain, depression, emotional problems, anxiety and many stress-related problems – frequently underlie insomnia, so it's no surprise that the therapy can also be very helpful in the treatment of insomnia itself.

CRYSTAL THERAPY

Here I must digress to tell a little story. Until a few years ago, like many people, I was unaware of the power of crystals. Then I was asked by the BBC to take part in a series of radio programs on complementary therapies. We drew up a list of those therapies that we wanted to cover and, since a friend of mine had recently introduced me to a crystal therapist, I thought we'd include her in the series.

Each program took the same format – the therapist would come to the studio and demonstrate his or her skills on a member of our team who had volunteered. On this occasion, Janet, the crystal healer, asked the volunteer, Barry, to lie down on the couch while she surrounded him with various crystals. No sooner had she started to do this than the producer's voice came in over the intercom: "What's going on in there? All the dials in here are going berserk!"

Apparently all the dials used to assess sound quality started oscillating wildly – and then stopped working completely. And so they remained until the end of the session when, once the crystals had been put away, they started to work normally again. Fortunately the team in the control room were experienced enough to be able to record the session adequately, even though they were "flying blind".

I tell this story to show how powerful crystals can be. I've discovered since then that you have to be very careful about putting crystals near any electrical equipment, especially computers. And not only do crystals affect the things around them but they themselves are affected by tensions and stresses in their surroundings. A practitioner I knew used to keep a large piece of rose quartz on his desk. His patients included a lot of people who were in pain and in distress – and one day the rose quartz just shattered into pieces. He later discovered that he should have washed it frequently and left it in sunlight to cleanse it of the energies that it had picked up from his patients.

If you are fortunate enough to have a really good crystal store in your neighborhood, you could ask for advice on which stones might benefit you. However, there are some shops that sell crystals more as decorative items than for their intrinsic powers, so you have to be careful. Since the best place to put stones to treat insomnia is under your pillow, you only need to buy small ones. You could also try carrying them round in your pocket during the day. Most of the crystals listed here are also available as crystal essences from companies such as Crystal Herbs Ltd.

(http://www.crystalherbs.com/)   Essences are prepared in a similar way to the Bach flower remedies - in other words, they contain the energies rather than the actual substance of the crystals.

The majority of the crystals listed here are widely available. However, you may have to visit a specialist crystal store to find cerussite, charoite, schalenblende and tourmaline. Lapis lazuli and schalenblende tend to be more expensive than the other crystals listed.

- **Amethyst** can take several forms, such as a single point, a cluster of crystals or a geode - a hollow rock with crystals growing inside. Its colour can vary and can be any shade between pale violet and deep purple. It is useful in the treatment of insomnia, particularly when this is in part or in whole due to your mind being unable to quieten down. It can also help to prevent recurrent nightmares. For the first few nights on which you use it, you may find that you dream more (or more vividly) but, after this, your sleep should become deeper, calmer and more refreshing.

  In addition to its value in treating insomnia, amethyst can help to disperse emotions such as anger, fear, anxiety and grief. It also relieves tension headaches, digestive disorders and may help to alleviate continual tiredness.

- **Aventurine** comes in a variety of colours, ranging from gray, though yellow, brown and blue to green. The commonest variety is green. It has shiny specks in it and is often sold as a tumbled (polished) stone

Aventurine promotes relaxation and so makes it easier to get to sleep. It may also relieve pain, stiffness, and anxiety, calm anger and annoyance, reduce allergy symptoms and alleviate migraine. Like amethyst, aventurine can stimulate dreaming.

- **Cerussite** can take the form of translucent white or yellow crystals, or a more granular grey. It is useful for treating insomnia, particularly where this has resulted from illness. It can also help to prevent nightmares and, because it can help you to adjust to a new situation, can be used to treat jet lag. It also helps to reduce tension and anxiety.

- **Blue chacedony** can have patterns of bands or whorls, depending on how it has been cut, and may be sold as a polished stone. It can help to prevent nightmares and promotes both relaxation and a feeling of optimism. It reduces both stress and feelings of self-doubt and can relieve symptoms brought about by a change in the weather. In particular, since it has a cooling effect, it may be useful if insomnia is being made worse by hot weather.

- **Charoite** is a mixture of mottled grey, pink, violet and purple, and is frequently sold as a polished stone. It can encourage deep, peaceful, refreshing sleep and, while it can prevent nightmares, it can also promote powerful and creative dreams.

It can also relieve cramp, headache and other aches and pains, so may be useful when insomnia is associated with menstrual cramps or painful conditions such as arthritis. It also helps to reduce the stress caused by major life changes by alleviating fear and anxiety and can be valuable when there is emotional turmoil by helping to put things in perspective.

- **Chrysoprase** is opaque and can be either apple green or lemon. It is helpful for mental and physical exhaustion, are calming and make it easier to drift off to sleep. It can help to reduce recurrent unpleasant images and nightmares and can give an feeling of security. It also helps to ease grief. Among its actions on the physical body, it can help to alleviate skin diseases and can balance hormones. It can be useful, therefore, when insomnia is associated with eczema or other itchy conditions or when it occurs as a result of PMS or menopausal changes.

- **Golden aragonite** is a beautiful translucent golden brown and may take the form of a little cluster of crystals, all pointing in different directions. It is particularly useful in reducing restlessness, and muscle twitching and spasm. It may therefore be helpful in reducing symptoms of restless leg syndrome and night-time muscle cramps. It has a calming effect and can also help to relieve pain, so may have a role when pain is preventing sleep.

- **Hematite** can be black, grey, red or reddish brown. It may be helpful in the treatment of insomnia which is associated with anxiety, stress or pain in the muscles or joints. It can also help to prevent night-time cramps in the legs.

  Hematite should only be used for short periods at a time and should never be put near inflamed skin, since it can cause increased irritation.

- **Howlite** can be white, green or blue and has a marbled appearance. It has a calming action and so can help when insomnia is due to fierce emotions or an overactive mind.

- **Lapis lazuli** literally means 'blue stone'. It is a rich, deep blue, speckled with gold and, during the Renaissance was crushed to make a pigment which was often used to paint the robes of the Virgin Mary. As well as being helpful in treating insomnia, it can relieve headaches, migraine and other pain, reduce inflammation and dispel anger which has been suppressed.

- **Lepidolite** ranges in colour from pink to purple. It can calm the mind, relieve stress and tension and reduce exhaustion, helping you to get to sleep and stay asleep through the night. It can also relieve neuralgia and pain in the joints and muscles. It may be particularly helpful where insomnia is associated with menopausal symptoms.

- **Magnesite** can be white, grey, yellow or brown, with either a 'knobbly' or a marbled appearance. It is an easily obtainable crystal that has a calming effect and can reduce fear and emotional stress. It can also act as a muscle relaxant and can ease headaches and migraine as well as menstrual and intestinal cramps.

- **Moonstone**: Ranging in colour from white to pale brown, and with a blue shimmer, moonstone is easily obtainable. It is particularly helpful for insomnia that has been precipitated by hormonal disturbances at the menopause, during or immediately after pregnancy, or associated with PMS. It reduces stress and may help to prevent sleepwalking where this has been a problem.

- **Muscovite** can be a variety of colours - pink, grey, brown, green, violet, yellow, red or white. As well as helping to relieve insomnia, it can have a beneficial effect on allergies and can alleviate self-doubt, anger and nervous stress.

- **Rose quartz**: Known as the crystal of love and peace, this lovely pink stone has a calming and relaxing effect. It can reduce emotional pain, worry, anxiety and grief.

- **Schalenblende**: Yellowish-brown, with bands of silver-grey, schalenblende is a beautiful crystal. It can relieve exhaustion, reduce fear and calm the mind, stopping thoughts from going round and round endlessly, allowing sleep to become possible.

- **Tourmaline** comes in a a number of different colours. The blue variety can help to prevent both nightmares and night sweats. It can also alleviate sadness and help to unblock emotions which have been bottled up.

To keep a crystal in perfect condition, you should cleanse it from time to time. Most crystals can be soaked in cold water in which a handful of sea salt has been dissolved. But this can damage angelite and some other crystals. Other methods include leaving the stone in strong sunlight (although this may bleach some colored stones, particularly rose quartz), burying it in the earth or leaving it next to a strongly growing plant. Or you can leave it for a while on top of an amethyst cluster which, itself, has cleansing properties and will rarely need cleaning. If in doubt, ask your crystal store for advice.

EFT (EMOTIONAL FREEDOM TECHNIQUE)

This is a relatively new therapy, developed in the last two decades of the twentieth century. It originated in the work of Dr. Roger Callaghan, a clinical psychologist who discovered that tapping certain points on the major acupuncture meridians could produce startling results in the treatment of psychological problems. He developed this further, using specific sequences of points to relate to different problems, and named the technique Thought Field Therapy (TFT).

An engineer, Gary Craig, who had been working with Neuro-Linguistic Programming (NLP) for some years, trained with Dr. Callaghan and, refining the technique still further, named his new system Emotional Freedom Technique. Because all the acupuncture meridians are interlinked, with energy flowing around them in a 24 hour cycle, Craig figured that if a blockage was removed from one meridian, it would automatically clear all the meridians. In the method that he devised only 14 points are used. These are tapped in no particular sequence while the patients focus on the problems that are troubling them.

EFT is now used for a wide range of psychological and psychosomatic problems. (It's important to note that "psychosomatic" does not mean "imaginary" but describes real physical problems that are made worse by stress, emotion, anxiety or other nervous conditions.) It is frequently used to treat addictions, phobias, anxiety, depression, migraine, pain, panic attacks, post traumatic stress, nightmares and insomnia. There are now practitioners in the UK as well as in many parts of North America.

HERBALISM (PHYTOTHERAPY)

Western herbalism

As one of the oldest therapies known to humankind, herbalism has a long tradition of effective treatment. In fact, some of its prescriptions have been so effective that modern orthodox drugs have been based on them. Probably the best known of these is digoxin used for treating heart failure. Centuries before it was extracted and synthesized by the pharmaceutical companies, digoxin in its "raw" form of digitalis, or foxglove, was being used by herbalists to treat the same condition.

When scientists investigate a herbal substance, they will try to extract the 'active principle' which they can then synthesize. They say that, in this way, they are developing a 'purer' form of the original herbal remedy, so that it can be prescribed in precise amounts. But herbalists always use the whole of the plant (or part of the plant, such as the root) because they believe that the active principle is, in its natural form, balanced by other components of the plant which, although not active in themselves, contribute to the efficacy of the remedy. This balance is more important, they believe, than knowing how much of each component is being prescribed to the nearest microgram.

However, because they do contain active chemical elements, herbs can be harmful if incorrectly used, unlike some other complementary therapies. If you intend to self-treat, you should use only those herbs that are widely available in health stores and you should never exceed the prescribed dose. If you are taking any medications, you should not try any herbal remedies without first talking to your physician. As with any therapy, the best results are likely to be achieved from consulting a qualified practitioner.

There are four classes of herbs that may be used to treat insomnia: hypnotics (which induce sleepiness), nervine relaxants (which relax the nervous system), antispasmodics (which relax the muscles) and nervine tonics (which strengthen the nervous system and are used when insomnia is associated with nervous exhaustion). A fifth class, adaptogens, which is useful for relieving stress, should only be taken during the day because these herbs (which include Korean, American and Siberian ginseng) also have a stimulant quality which may prevent sleep. Some plants fall into two or more classes.

There are numerous books and websites that recommend herbal preparations (usually in the form of teas) for various ailments. But a glance at several of these will show you that they're not all telling you the same thing. Look up "insomnia" in one and you will be told chamomile, deadnettle, hawthorn, lady's mantle or St. John's wort. Another will suggest basil, California poppy, cowslip, hops or rosemary. A third will tell you to use corydalis, kava kava, passion flower, tarragon or valerian. By the time you get to the fourth, your head is swimming and you don't know who to believe or what to try. The problem is that, while some of these herbs are true soporifics, others are useful for treating insomnia which is due, for example, to anxiety or restlessness or muscular pain, and are used to treat the underlying cause rather than the insomnia itself. The simplest solution is to consult a qualified herbalist.

However, if you do want to try self-treatment, make sure that the remedies come from a reputable herbal pharmacy or manufacturer and never exceed the recommended dosage since certain herbs can be toxic in large amounts. And unless you buy a ready-made preparation which contains several herbs, only use one herb at a time. This way you will be able to assess the effect of the herb more easily.

Herbs to treat insomnia

Of all the herbs that can be used to treat insomnia or aspects of insomnia, the following few are perhaps some of the most widely recommended.

- **California poppy:** a gentle hypnotic and antispasmodic, this herb also has analgesic (pain-killing) properties but, unlike its relative, the opium poppy, it's not a narcotic. For a night-time drink, pour a cup of boiling water onto 1 or 2 teaspoons of the dried herb and leave it to infuse for about ten minutes. Or take between 1 and 4 ml of the tincture at bedtime.

- **hops:** a hypnotic and antispasmodic, the sedative properties of hops were realized from very early times because hop pickers seem to tire very easily. It is also used as a treatment for acid indigestion, restlessness and irritability. It's particularly useful for insomnia which is caused by anxiety or worry. In many cases the smell of hops can alleviate a headache although prolonged contact with hops or an excessive intake can, in fact, cause a headache. Hops are also helpful for treating menopausal problems and, in particular, sleep problems made worse by hot flashes.

For a night-time drink, put 1 or 2 teaspoons of fresh, dried or freeze-dried hops in a cup of boiling water and leave to soak for about 5 minutes. Or 1 to 4 ml of the tincture can be taken up to three times a day. Another use for hops is to put them in a "sleep pillow" which will release its fragrance whenever you turn your head. Other herbs that may be used together with hops in a pillow are catnip leaves and linden flowers. Dried hops shouldn't be kept for too long because their properties fade quite quickly. Because they have an estrogenic effect, they should be used only very sparingly during pregnancy. And they should never be used by anyone suffering from depression as they can make the condition worse.

- **Jamaica dogwood** – this is a powerful sedative which is useful in the treatment of neuralgia, migraine and other painful conditions and in insomnia particularly when this is being caused by worry, anxiety or pain. Some books suggest that it is especially useful for treating children and the elderly. Other indications for its use are arthritis and cough. Herbalists may combine it with hops and valerian to treat insomnia.

For a night-time drink, put a teaspoonful of the root in a cup of water, bring it to the boil and simmer gently for 10 to 15 minutes. Or take 1 to 2 ml of the tincture before bedtime. The recommended dose should never be exceeded as larger quantities can be toxic. Some herbalists recommend that it should only be used under the supervision of a qualified therapist.

- Just in passing, I'll mention **lady's slipper** which, because it's now fairly scarce and therefore expensive, is not often used nowadays. But it has a long history in North America, since the native Americans used a boiled extract to calm the nerves and early settlers used it as a substitute for valerian, which they had used in Europe. Today its main claim to fame seems to be as the State flower of Minnesota, while in the UK it's a protected species so that it's illegal to pick it or dig it up when it's growing in the wild. Although it's not a herb that's readily available for self-help use, it is still used occasionally by herbalists to treat insomnia (particularly when this is due to the mind going round and round), anxiety, restlessness, irritability, neuralgia and menopausal depression. One standard textbook describes it as "favoring mental tranquillity". It is also indicated for the treatment of muscle twitches, so it may be useful when insomnia is associated with RLS or PLMS.

- **passion flower** (passiflora):   a hypnotic and antispasmodic, this herb is said to give a feeling of well being and to reduce anxiety. Some herbalists consider it to be the remedy of choice for long-standing insomnia, particularly when associated with neuralgic pain or with asthma. However, it may be less effective when the patient is suffering from arthritic or other types of pain although it is a herb that some textbooks recommend as specifically for insomnia in the elderly. Others recommend it for insomnia due to worry or overwork. (Although the textbooks also suggest this herb as a treatment for sleeplessness in children, you should never give a child a herbal remedy – other than a commercial preparation that clearly states that it is suitable for children – except on the advice of a qualified herbalist.)

One standard textbook describes passion flower as inducing "a quiet, peaceful slumber, undisturbed by any unpleasantness, and the patient awakens calm and refreshed". You may, however, need to take it for a few days before you start to feel the full benefit. It's also effective against muscle spasms and so may be useful in the treatment of RLS and PLMS. Although usually free of side effects, it may cause nausea, in which case it should be discontinued. One authority advises against taking the herb if you have a flushed face or a heavily coated tongue as the action will not be satisfactory.

Passion flower shouldn't be taken by people who are on MAOI antidepressants as it can reduce their effect. To make a bedtime drink, pour a cup of boiling water onto half a teaspoon of the dried herb.

- **St. John's wort**: this is a nervine tonic which is used to treat tension, anxiety, insomnia and depression, especially when these are associated with the menopause. It also lowers the blood pressure. Its effects in mild to moderate depression have been confirmed by scientific clinical trials. American studies have found that its effect is increased when taken together with Ginkgo biloba, but this combination should only be taken on the advice of a herbalist or physician, not as a self-help remedy. St. John's wort is not without side effects – it makes skin more light sensitive, so people with fair skins should avoid exposure to ultraviolet light – primarily strong sunlight and tanning beds. People taking this herb should also avoid red wine, cheese, yeast and pickled herring since these can cause unpleasant reactions. However, menopausal women who are prepared to abide by these restrictions may find it an ideal remedy for their symptoms. The dose is 500mg a day of the extract with meals, or 1 to 2 ml of the tincture three times a day. An infusion (which can also be taken three times a day) can be made by pouring a cup of boiling water onto 1 to 2 teaspoons of the dried herb and leaving it for 10 to 14 minutes.

- **skullcap:** a hypnotic, antispasmodic and nervine tonic, this herb was used by physicians in the nineteenth century to treat conditions that we now call fibromyalgia and chronic fatigue syndrome. Its action in controlling muscle spasm makes it a good choice where insomnia is caused or aggravated by RLS or PLMS. It is also effective for nervous tension, restlessness and premenstrual tension and where sleep is being disturbed by nightmares. It seems not to have any side effects. An infusion can be made by pouring a cup of boiling water onto 1 or 2 teaspoons of the dried herb and leaving it for 10 to 15 minutes before drinking. This can be taken as a bedtime drink or three times a day as a mild sedative. Skullcap can also be taken in tincture form (2 to 4 ml three times a day) or put in a sleep pillow.

- **valerian:** a hypnotic and antispasmodic and perhaps the most widely researched of any herbal insomnia treatment, it was known to be a sedative by the ancient Romans and has been used ever since. Not only does it improve your ability to fall asleep but it also improves the quality of sleep.

One leading teacher of herbalism, David L. Hoffmann, says of valerian "As one of the best gentle and harmless herbal sleeping remedies, it enhances the natural body process of slipping into sleep and making the stresses of the day recede. For people who do not need as much sleep as they once did, it also eases lying awake in bed, ensuring that it becomes a restful and relaxing experience."

Although it has been recognized and approved by the United States FDA, valerian can be mildly habit forming and higher doses may become necessary to achieve the same effect. For this reason it should only be taken for short periods (no more than a month) and then tailed off, or else should be taken just occasionally as needed unless otherwise prescribed by a herbalist or physician. It can be taken as a tincture - the dose is 2.5 to 5 ml about an hour before bedtime – start with the lower dose and increase gradually over a period of a week or so until you achieve the best dose to give you a good night's sleep. Occasionally doses up to 10 ml are necessary to achieve the desired effect but, although side effects are unlikely, you should consult a herbalist or herbal pharmacist before taking over 5 ml. The herb can also be taken as an infusion, either by using boiling water on two teaspoons of the dried herb and drinking after 10 to 15 minutes or by soaking two teaspoons of the root in a glass of cold water for 8 to 10 hours.

Valerian shouldn't be taken by women who are pregnant or by anyone taking barbiturates. It doesn't impair your ability to drive or operate machinery but it's probably best to avoid alcohol if you are taking it regularly. As well as relieving insomnia, valerian is useful in the treatment of anxiety and emotional stress and can help to relax tense muscles.

HOMEOPATHY

A brief introduction

Modern homeopathy was developed in the late 18th century by the German, Samuel Hahnemann. Like Dr. Edward Bach (whose flower remedies were discussed above), Franz Mesmer the "Father" of hypnotherapy and Dr. Albert Abrams the discoverer of radionics, Hahnemann was a well qualified and highly respected orthodox physician whose visionary ideals led him to look for other ways in which he could help his patients.

Hahnemann's idea of "like cures like" remains the basis of homeopathy today: a substance which, when taken by a healthy person, will produce certain symptoms will, if given to someone who has those same symptoms as the result of a disease, cure them. For example, give quinine in sufficient quantity to a healthy person and they will develop a yellowing of the skin, nausea and a fever – all of which are symptoms of malaria. But in orthodox medicine quinine has long been used to treat malaria.

Hahnemann experimented with a number of substances in this way and found that his thesis worked in every case. But some of these substances were toxic, so he diluted them. And what he found was that, when the concentration of the substance was reduced and the dilution was performed in a particular way (called "potentization"), the resultant remedy became *more* effective the more dilute it became. Nowadays the strongest (and therefore the least powerful) of the remedies commonly used is a 6c – which has been diluted one in a hundred six times. Now it doesn't need a mathematician to work out that this means that there's very little – if any – of the original substance left. And this is one reason why skeptics have attacked homeopathy and said that it only works because of the placebo effect – in other words because the patient believes it will.

However, when you look at it closely, this argument doesn't wash. Many more patients do well with homeopathy than can be accounted for by the placebo effect (which is generally said to be around 30 per cent of those treated, although recent scientific papers have suggested that it might be considerably lower than this). In addition, a large number of double blind trials have shown that homeopathy can produce significant benefits. And, of course, the fact that (like other complementary therapies) it works well on animals, small children and people in comas, for whom the placebo effect cannot possibly be an influence, offers additional evidence of its value.

How the effect of high dilution works, however, is still unclear. Recent theories have suggested that the "energy" of the substance is transferred to the diluting water, something that may link in to discoveries in the field of quantum physics. But, however it works, the dilution means that homeopathic remedies are far safer than conventional drugs.

Since Hahnemann's time, many more remedies have been developed by using his own method of "proving". A substance is given over a period of time to a group of healthy people and the symptoms that they develop are recorded and form the "symptom picture" for that remedy. There are now well over 2000 remedies available to the homeopath and many of these have large and complex symptom pictures.

The skill of the homeopath is to match the remedy to the patient because, the closer the match, the more likely is the prospect of a cure. And the match involves not just the symptoms of the current problem but also everything about the patient – including their sleeping habits, eating habits, likes, dislikes and personality. So it is for this reason that homeopathy may not be successful as a self-help treatment other than as a first-aid measure. While Arnica, for example, is almost invariably the treatment of choice for shock and injury (especially bruising) and Apis for bee and wasp stings, more complex conditions require a much more detailed knowledge of the remedies available in order to achieve the closest possible match.

And so, although it is possible to self-treat for insomnia, you are more likely to get good results if you consult a qualified homeopath. If you do want to treat yourself, however, choose the remedy which most closely matches your symptoms and take a single tablet (dissolved under the tongue) at bedtime for about a week. If after that time it hasn't helped, stop taking it because to continue will run the risk of eventually proving it – developing the symptoms associated with that substance. In most health stores only the lowest potency (6c) is available but 12c or 30c are quite safe for self-treatment. (Homeopaths have a much wider range of potencies available, the higher potencies being usually more effective for chronic conditions.)

Homeopathic remedies

Of the numerous remedies that might be used to treat insomnia, the following are, perhaps, some of the most obvious. You don't need to be suffering from all the symptoms listed for a remedy to be the right one for you. If it contains your most striking or troublesome symptoms, there is a good chance that it will help.

- **Aconitum apellus**: try this one if you become fearful or agitated while you're drifting off to sleep and then have vivid and frightening dreams or if you're woken up by panic attacks. Aconitum can also be useful if your insomnia has occurred as the result of an illness.

- **Arnica**: as well as being a valuable first aid remedy for injury, arnica may be useful when insomnia is due to physical overwork and your body is aching or you just can't get comfortable and the bed feels too hard. It's also worth trying if you have jet lag.

- **Arsenicum album**: the arsenicum "type" tends to be a perfectionist who often becomes anxious about small details, gets thirsty but only sips water, feels cold and may prefer to sleep propped up. Try Arsenicum if you're mentally and physically restless despite being very tired or even exhausted, or if you get anxious at night and your sleep is disturbed by dreams that are full of fear and insecurity.

- **Calcarea phosphorica (Calc. phos.)**: may help if you have aching joints or tense muscles in your neck and shoulders, if you lie awake for ages feeling upset and irritable and, in the morning, feel tired and weak and have difficulty waking up.

- **Chamomilla:** if your insomnia is due to pain or anger or is the result of taking drugs (of any sort – prescribed, over-the-counter or illegal), if you tend to be irritable and argumentative, if you're drowsy during the day but find it hard to sleep before about 2am and if you have frightening dreams, then Chamomilla may be the remedy of choice. Ask your partner if you moan while you're asleep and if your eyes look as though they're half open – these are both indications for Chamomilla.   It's also helpful when sleeplessness is due to having drunk too much coffee.

- **Cocculus:** try this if you're exhausted as the result of sleep deprivation over a long period (perhaps because you've been looking after a baby or a sick relative or because you've had persistent worries keeping you awake) but you're still unable to sleep even though conditions have changed. Other indicators for taking Cocculus are associated weakness, dizziness, difficulty thinking straight, irritability and a tendency to cry easily. This remedy may also be helpful for jet lag.

- **Coffea cruda:** this is the homeopathic remedy prepared from coffee and so if it's too much coffee that's keeping you awake, you could try this, although cutting down on your coffee intake might be more sensible. Coffea may also be the right remedy for you if you can't sleep because your mind's working overtime (the thoughts don't have to be stressful ones – they can be happy and exciting) and if you sleep only lightly, wake at the slightest sound, have vivid dreams, and tend to wake around 4am after which you can't get to sleep again. Coffea is also helpful when insomnia occurs around the time of the menopause or after pregnancy.

- **Gelsemium (Gels.):** if you've been studying very hard, you're exhausted and you're worried about what the future holds, you could try Gelsemium. Despite having to study, you're likely to feel mentally sluggish and may fall asleep after your evening meal or while you're studying but you then find you can't get to sleep after going to bed and you have bad dreams in the early hours of the morning. Gelsemium may also be useful when insomnia is associated with pregnancy or with heavy smoking.

- **Hyoscyamus:** if your sleeplessness is due to excitement, anger, worries about your business or distress following an unhappy love affair, if you're restless and find it difficult to sleep between midnight and dawn even though you're sleepy during the day, and if you tend to wake with a start, this may be the remedy for you. Ask your partner if you mutter or laugh while you're asleep as these are further indications for using Hyoscyamus.

- **Ignatia:** if an emotional upset (particularly as a result of breaking up with someone you love), bad news, worry, depression, anger or a back injury lies at the root of your insomnia, if you're a sensitive and nervous person who sighs and yawns a lot, if your moods are very changeable and if you sleep lightly and tend to have long or repetitive nightmares, you could try Ignatia. It's also worth a try if you've been diagnosed as having RLS or PLMS because the symptom picture of Ignatia includes muscle twitching and itching and muscle spasms while sleeping.

- **Kali phosphoricum (Kali phos.):** this may be suitable if you're suffering from mental strain or from nervous exhaustion due to overwork or if you're recovering from a long illness. Other indicators would be that you feel very weak, you're irritable, depressed and anxious and you wake with a sinking feeling in your stomach. It may be helpful in RLS because Kali phos. patients often have "fidgety feet".

- **Lachesis** is particularly indicated for sleep problems that occur around the time of the menopause. Try it if, just as you're dropping off to sleep, you get a sense of suffocation in your throat or you feel as though the bed's swaying, especially if these symptoms make you dread going to bed or going to sleep. Other indicators for this remedy are a tendency to hold your breath while you're falling asleep, night sweats, and waking up feeling anxious and unwell.

- **Lycopodium:** if you don't remember your dreams and sometimes wonder if you've slept at all, you may need Lycopodium. Your insomnia may originally have been due to worry or to digestive problems and you may wake up in the night feeling very hungry. You may also lack confidence in yourself although the chances are that you're very capable.

- **Nux vomica:** if you've been overindulging – in food, alcohol or even drugs – or if you've been over-exerting yourself – physically or mentally - and you can't sleep as a result, Nux vomica may help. It may also be helpful if you've "tried everything" for your insomnia and nothing has helped. Other indications are sleeping lightly and waking early (typically at 3 am), then lying awake for hours, possibly falling into a heavy sleep at daybreak, and getting up feeling tense, tired and irritable. You're also likely to be irritable and tense during the day, sensitive to noise, light and smells, and you may be a perfectionist or a workaholic – or both! Nux vomica is also helpful when insomnia is being caused by medications or is the result of coming off tranquilizers or sedatives.

- **Pulsatilla:** try this if you're restless when you first go to bed, feel first hot and then cold, find it hard to sleep in a warm room, sleep with your arms above your head, have anxious or vivid dreams and night sweats and wake early with your mind racing, and if your insomnia is aggravated by eating rich food (particularly pork or ice cream) and sometimes your lack of sleep makes you cry.

- **Sepia:** if you have difficulty falling asleep and then wake up early feeling unrefreshed, you're exhausted and depressed as a result of overwork or mental stress, if you tend to be irritable and sleepy during the day, suffer from night sweats and get headaches, nausea and dizziness as a result of being tired, try Sepia.

- **Sulphur:** may be indicated if you're being kept awake by itching or by ideas going round and round in your mind, or if you feel very hot in bed (especially your feet) and need to throw off the covers or stick your feet out of the bed, if you lie awake between 2am and 5am and then sleep late, if you're wakened by the slightest noise, have vivid nightmares and tend to be irritable and anxious.

- **Thuja:** if you wake early feeling unrefreshed and if the parts of your body that you've been lying on are painful you might try Thuja. Other indications are talking in your sleep and anxious dreams.

- Zincum metallicum is another remedy that may be indicated in the treatment of RLS. The symptom picture includes having trouble relaxing, nervousness, nervous exhaustion, a constant need to move the legs and arms even during the day, a total inability to lie still in bed, and jerky movements as you fall asleep.

HYPNOTHERAPY

We all know what hypnosis is . . . we see it on TV and in the movies . . quite often it's done by a guy swinging a watch in front of someone's eyes and saying (usually in a foreign accent) "You are falling asleep . ."

And we've seen 'reality' shows where the subjects have been made to do whatever the hypnotist tells them. As a result, you may, quite reasonably, be a bit dubious about hypnotism which looks as though it consists of someone "taking over your mind" and making you do things, possibly against your will. This idea may be reinforced by the fact that hypnotherapy can help people to give up smoking – giving the impression that they are *made* to stop. So let me make it clear straight away that this view of hypnosis is completely inaccurate.

But why, then, does it *look* as though this is true? Well, obviously, in a movie, you can make anything look true – a fifty foot high gorilla or a man in a cape flying over the Empire State Building. And, just like a movie, a stage hypnotist is providing entertainment, not realism. So, to begin with he'll usually start by getting the audience to play some games, which are actually tests to see who will be a good hypnotic subject. Then, once everyone's in a party mood and ready to join in the show, he'll pick out a number of those who look as though they're likely subjects and ask them to come up on stage. Anyone who doesn't want to join in will probably refuse at this point so the chances are that he'll now have a group of people on stage who, as long as he doesn't ask them to do anything completely against their principles (like taking their clothes off) will be happy to co-operate.

This is not to say, however, that stage hypnosis is always safe – people may be profoundly embarrassed or distressed afterwards by some of the silly things they've been asked to do. And certainly the trick that some hypnotists do of making someone go rigid, lying them across the top of two chairs and then asking someone else to stand on them can be very dangerous. But, since the subject is unlikely to realize the dangers of going rigid, he or she will probably acquiesce. This is not a case of the hypnotist taking over the subject's mind – just a case of the subject's subconscious mind not realizing that there is a good reason to refuse to comply.

And what about smoking? Well, you hear a lot about people who have given up with the help of hypnosis – but there are also a lot of people who have had hypnosis and *haven't* given up. They're the ones who don't really want to give up – who are trying hypnosis because their partner or child or parent or physician wants them to give up or because it makes financial sense or because they're worried about the harm it will do their health. But deep down, they like smoking and they don't *want* to give up. So they won't.

This, then, is the key to hypnotherapy. The way it acts is to enable you to do things that you really want to do, even if you think it may be impossible. It has a very good record in treating all manner of problems from skin conditions (eczema, psoriasis) to migraine and even epilepsy. It can help children to stop bed-wetting, women to go through childbirth and insomniacs to sleep.

In order for hypnosis to work, the subject has to be willing to accept the suggestions given while he (or she) is in trance. Now, insomniacs are likely to be more than happy to take on board suggestions that will give them a good night's sleep, so one would imagine that the therapy would be successful 100 per cent of the time. But, unfortunately, it isn't. One of the reasons for this this lies in what I've already touched on in regard to stage hypnosis – the fact that some people are better subjects than others, more likely to go into hypnosis and more susceptible to suggestion.

Some people just can't be hypnotized. There are two reasons for this – either they are resisting or else they want to be hypnotized so much that they are "willing themselves" to go under – which is rather like willing yourself to go to sleep. It doesn't work. If you are able to take a relaxed attitude and just let it happen when the therapist is inducing hypnosis, then you are far more likely to go into a trance. But that's not always easy if you are desperate for the therapy to work. For this reason, it may be helpful to try something such as meditation (described in a section later on) in order to attain this relaxed attitude before seeing a hypnotherapist.

It may seem unlikely that anyone who is visiting a therapist for treatment will actively resist that treatment, but it's possible to do this without realizing it. It's said that people such as actors, soldiers and nurses are likely to be good subjects because they are used to doing what they are told. But the people who give the orders - the directors, drill sergeants and doctors – are less likely to be easily hypnotized.

However, if you are one of those people who goes easily into a hypnotic trance, then you may find this a very useful therapy. I should say a word here about the trance itself. Once again, many people have the wrong impression, believing that being in hypnosis is like being asleep and that the subject can remember nothing afterwards of what went on. And because hypnosis is *not* like this, many hypnotherapy patients refuse to believe after the first session that they have actually been hypnotized – until, of course, the therapy starts to work.

One simple way of explaining the difference between states of consciousness is to look at how the subject reacts to outside stimuli. Imagine that you are sitting in a room with a couple of friends. You have your eyes shut but you are listening to them talk. Suddenly they start to discuss something that's of interest to you – you'll probably open your eyes and join in the conversation. If you were in a light trance in similar circumstances, you would listen to what they were saying but wouldn't want to join in. If you were in a deep trance, you'd *hear* what they were saying but you wouldn't actively listen.

Occasionally, a patient who goes into a very deep trance will not remember what has happened during the session but this is uncommon, not least because a very deep trance is unnecessary for treating most conditions. Sometimes, if the patient has been regressed – when hypnosis is used with psychotherapy – distressing memories may be unearthed. Very often, just bringing them out under hypnosis is enough to dispel the trauma surrounding them. The usual procedure is for the hypnotherapist to tell the patient, while still in the trance, that he or she will forget what has emerged during the session *until such time as the conscious mind is strong enough to cope with it*. This usually results in the memory coming through gradually at a later date in a far less traumatic way. I should also point out here that, even if you do go into a fairly deep trance, you are still in control and can wake yourself up at any time.

But what about insomnia? Well, there are two reasons why I've gone into the whys and wherefores of the therapy itself in such depth. The first has been to offer reassurance that hypnosis is not as frightening as it may sometimes be made to appear. And the second is to emphasize that, although in trained hands hypnosis is safe and effective, in untrained hands it can sometimes be harmful. If you are seeing a hypnotherapist to try to give up smoking, as long as he has had a basic training, you are unlikely to come to any harm. But for anything that requires a psychotherapeutic approach (and this may well include insomnia) it is wisest to consult a hypnotherapist who is either a physician or a psychotherapist.

And what can you expect from hypnotherapy? Well, in the treatment of insomnia it can be used in two ways. The first is as a relaxation technique. Because, when you get down to it, hypnosis is really just an extremely deep form of relaxation. If you are a good subject and go easily into a trance, it is likely that the therapist will give you certain suggestions about how relaxed you will feel before bedtime and how easily you will settle down once you are in bed.

You may also be taught self-hypnosis. This can be very useful because it means that, when you put out the light and close your eyes, instead of just lying waiting to go to sleep, you can put yourself into a hypnotic trance from which you will drift into a normal sleep. The second way in which hypnosis can be used is to help you to find the causes of your insomnia. This can be especially valuable when particular stresses have precipitated your sleep problems. However, this form of therapy can take some time before it is effective, although it is likely to have lasting effects.

Because I am an experienced hypnotherapist, I have made a 15 minute hypnosis mp3 which I am giving away free to anyone who has bought this book. It will allow you to experience a light hypnotic trance in the comfort of your own home and it offers suggestions to help you sleep better. To get your copy, please go to:

http://sphinxhouse.com/get-your-free-hypnotherapy-mp3/

MEDITATION AND VISUALIZATION

A brief introduction

Although most forms of meditation have spiritual associations, they can also be used very successfully as a form of relaxation therapy. From a spiritual point of view, the purpose of the basic meditation practice (whether it is a form of breathing or the repetition of a mantra or the visualization of a particular shape or scene) is to focus and clarify the mind so that it becomes open and able to receive wisdom, inspiration or enlightenment. Now, if the mind is truly focused, there is no room for extraneous thoughts, so this can be a powerful way of calming the mind. However, it may take a great deal of practice.

The two forms of meditation that are, perhaps, the most suitable for the treatment of insomnia are breathing techniques such as the Buddhist anapanasati (or mindfulness of breathing) or the repetition of a mantra.

Anapanasati (Mindfulness of Breathing)

In order to use this as a relaxation technique, it is necessary, first of all, to be comfortable. The actual position doesn't matter – you may be lying on your back or your side or even your front, if that's the position in which you most usually manage to fall asleep. You may have your arms by your sides or crossed or even above your head. Your legs can be bent or straight. What is important is that no part of your body feels strained.

Once you've found this position, become aware of your breathing. Don't try to change the rhythm or the rate or the depth. Just be aware of how you are breathing in and out. And then start counting the breaths, counting either the in-breaths or the out-breaths but not both. When you get to ten, start again at one. And while you are counting, keep your mind clear of all other thoughts. If you are distracted, just start again at one. And keep going . . .

The effectiveness of this technique in inducing sleep can be demonstrated by the frequency with which people who are using this as a meditation (rather than a relaxation) technique tend to fall asleep while using it if they happen to be tired. One of the jobs of the head monk in a Zen meditation hall is to make sure that the other monks stay awake!

It takes practice but, once it starts to work, you should find that it becomes more effective the more regularly you use it.

Mantras

A mantra is simply a word or phrase which is repeated over and over again in order to put the mind into a certain state. In some cases the goal is to arouse religious fervor or a sense of spiritual awareness. Life coaches teach mantras (often referred to as affirmations) to their clients as a way of building self-confidence.

Whereas some mantras may be several syllables or words long, a relaxation mantra needs to be short and easy to repeat in the mind without the necessity of having to remember something complicated. A single syllable may be used such as "mee" or "soo" which can be repeated in rhythm with the out-breaths. You can either repeat it out loud (if you sleep alone) or in your head.

Dr. Shen Hongxun, who teaches Taijiwuxigong (a form of exercise associated with spontaneous movement) and Buqi (a therapy based on it) has developed his own mantra, Menm Tshh, which will combat insomnia. To quote from his book *Spontaneous Movement for Health and Happiness*: "When you pronounce the sound 'Menm' , you breathe out while keeping the mouth closed . . . When you pronounce the sound "Tshh", you breathe out but you can have your mouth slightly opened . . In the beginning use a low but clear voice to recite the sound. The more you recite it the softer your voice becomes, the slower and the lower the sound is pronounced. After a while you become more and more relaxed; you are only slowly whispering the sound and you will fall asleep."

Visualization

One could say that visualization falls midway between meditation and hypnosis because it's a technique that's used by both. When it's used in a spiritual context in meditation, the visualization is likely to be of a religious object, person or deity. However, in hypnosis it's used as a relaxation technique, taking the hypnotized person deeper into the trance. And used by itself, even without a hypnotic induction, it can be a very valuable relaxation tool.

What's your favorite way of relaxing? Lying on a beach? Walking in the country? Sitting in a garden? Whatever it is, when you use visualization as a relaxation technique, you need to take this scene and make it even better. So, for example, if you choose lying on a beach, it's not just any beach that you picture in your mind. It's a deserted beach with fine white sand that stretches for miles, a clear deep blue sea with tiny waves breaking softly, sea birds calling up in the unclouded sky, a light breeze and warm sunshine, perhaps an umbrella to keep you cool. Try to hear the sound of the waves and of the birds, feel the warmth of the sun and the breeze on your skin . . .

Similarly, if you visualize yourself walking in the countryside, there must be no one else around – perhaps the odd rabbit or other small animal, a stream trickling over stones, glorious views, warm sunshine and a little breeze. . . And if you're in a garden, imagine beautiful flowers – try to smell their fragrance, hear the sound of a little fountain and birds singing in the trees . . . Whatever your scene, always to try incorporate all your senses into it – not just sight but the feel of the breeze and the sun, the smell of the sea or the flowers, the sound of the water and the birds. The more you can lose yourself in the scene, the more relaxed you will become and the more likely you are to fall asleep.

NUTRITION THERAPY AND SUPPLEMENTS

There are many ways in which the things we eat and drink can affect our sleeping patterns. Everyone knows that coffee can keep you awake because of its caffeine content. But many people drink hot chocolate at night without realizing that it, too, contains caffeine. And most people think that alcohol will help them sleep whereas, as was pointed out in the section on *Do's and Don'ts for a Good Night's Sleep*, it actually makes sleep lighter and more fragmented because it suppresses both deep sleep and REM sleep.

Serotonin

Serotonin, which was first identified in 1948, is a naturally occurring chemical that is found in the intestines, the brain and the blood. Its functions are still not fully understood but it is known to play a role in regulating sleep. When the serotonin level in the brain rises, we feel sleepy. So anything that raises or lowers the levels of serotonin in the brain will affect your ability to sleep.

The traditional idea of a hot milky drink at bedtime is a good one because milk contains the amino-acid **tryptophan** which the body turns first into **5-hydroxytryptophan** (5HTP) and then into serotonin (5-hydroxytryptomine or 5HT). Tryptophan is found in many foods. Those containing significant amounts include chocolate, oats, dates, bananas, yoghurt, cottage cheese, poultry, sunflower and pumpkin seeds, and peanuts. So a light snack containing any of these, eaten an hour or two before bedtime, may be beneficial.

However, the body cannot convert tryptophan into serotonin if larger amounts of two other amino-acids, phenylalanine and leucine, are present. Wholegrain wheat and rye breads both have a high ratio of phenylalanine and leucine to tryptophan and, while they are very unlikely in themselves to cause insomnia, it might be best to avoid eating them late at night. On the other hand, dates, bananas and papayas have a low ratio of phenylalanine and leucine to tryptophan and so make good late night snacks because the tryptophan is available to increase serotonin levels.

Carbohydrates also help our bodies to produce serotonin, so that a diet which is rich in starchy foods – such as fruit, pasta, rice, bread, cereals and potatoes – will be beneficial. It follows that a low carbohydrate diet (such as the Atkins diet) may cause disruption to sleep in susceptible individuals by lowering the serotonin level. So if you suffer from insomnia but want to lose weight, you might be better off trying a low fat diet (such as Patrick Holford's *30 day fat-burner diet*) which will be less likely to cause a drop in serotonin levels. However, it's important to emphasize that sugar and sugary foods, although they're carbohydrate, can cause sleep to be disturbed if eaten in the evening because they rapidly raise the blood sugar level, producing a burst of energy.

Both tryptophan and 5HTP are available as supplements. However, the value of tryptophan is debatable because, although it can shorten the length of time it takes to get to sleep, it may alter the pattern of sleep by reducing the time spent in REM. It should never be taken with antidepressants because it can interact with them, causing serious side effects.

Supplements of 5-HTP are probably more effective. Studies have shown that it will increase the amount of time spent in REM sleep (the part of the sleep cycle in which we dream) and in deep sleep. It won't increase the total time spent asleep but, by altering the pattern of sleep in this way, it makes it more restful and refreshing.

If you decide to try 5-HTP supplements, you should take 100mg 30 or 40 minutes before bedtime and continue with this dose for at least three days. If it isn't having the desired effect, you can increase it gradually to a maximum of 300mg, allowing at least three days each time to see whether the dose is working. Higher doses may cause disturbing dreams or nightmares, so you should always stick with the lowest effective dose. The conversion of 5-HTP into serotonin requires vitamin B3 (niacin) and magnesium, so you may want to take supplements of these as well.

Before taking 5-HTP, or any other supplements, check with your physician that they will not interact with any medication that you are on.

Vitamin and mineral supplements

As mentioned in section above, when 5-HTP is converted to serotonin in the body, it needs adequate levels of **vitamin B3** (niacin) and **magnesium** to perform the conversion. **Vitamins B3 and B6** can also help to ease anxiety while **B5** (pantothenic acid) can help alleviate the results of stress. The best sources of B vitamins are cereals and seeds.

Inositol, which is also a part of the B vitamin compound, enhances REM sleep.

Calcium, too, can have a beneficial effect on sleeping (another reason why the hot milky drink can be a sedative) but needs to be taken together with magnesium, in a ratio of 2:1. (This is the ratio found in Dolomite tablets, which should be available from health stores.) Not only can these two minerals help to induce sleep, but a deficiency can cause cramps in the legs during the night.

If you want to take individual supplements at bedtime, the following doses are recommended:

> 600mg calcium with 200mg magnesium.
> 100mg inositol.
> 50mg vitamin B6
> 500mg vitamin B3
> 25mg vitamin B12
> 100mg vitamin B5

However, you may feel that taking all these is a bit excessive. And, in fact, it's probably better just to take a high dose combination vitamin and mineral supplement which includes all these. In most cases this will consist of one tablet two or three times a day, so you can take the last dose half an hour or so before bedtime.

Food and drinks to avoid

We have already mentioned alcohol and caffeine-containing drinks (including not only coffee but also tea, chocolate and cola) under this heading.

Foods to avoid in the evening include cheese, chocolate, bacon and ham, sugar, eggplant, potatoes, spinach and tomatoes because these all contain tyramine which causes the body to release a chemical called norepinephrine which stimulates the brain.

Heavy, fatty meals should also be avoided in the evening because these are hard to digest.

Melatonin

As evening falls and it starts to get dark, the pineal gland in the brain begins to secrete the hormone melatonin in increasing amounts. This hormone acts as a stimulus to sleep, which means that constant bright light (which inhibits the secretion of melatonin) can prevent sleep. In recent times it has been discovered that it is the blue component of light which is especially involved in this. This makes sense – human beings have evolved in a way that the blue light of dawn wakes them up while the pink light of evening makes them feel sleepy. However, in the modern age, when we have electric lighting and, particularly, television (which emits a lot of blue light), the natural changes in light from day to night no longer affect us as they affected our ancestors.

Melatonin in tablet form is available as an over-the-counter supplement, but its usefulness in the treatment of insomnia is debatable. What has been found, though, is that it can be valuable in resetting the 'biological clock', whose disruption is the cause of jet lag. However, even here, only fifty per cent of those people who take it are likely to find it effective.

Some studies have found melatonin supplements to be helpful in inducing and maintaining sleep in both children and adults but, mostly, the indications seem to be that, while it may help you to fall asleep, it won't do much to keep you asleep throughout the night.

In addition, melatonin may have side effects – there have been isolated reports of it exacerbating depression and fatigue and causing constriction of the arteries that supply the heart. More commonly, it has been found to cause drowsiness, headache and even confusion the morning after taking it, and it can increase the incidence of vivid dreams and nightmares.

Because of the risk of side effects, it may be best to avoid melatonin supplements except as a first aid remedy for jet lag. And they should be avoided altogether by women who are pregnant or breast feeding, and by people with cancer, heart disease, high blood pressure, immune deficiency or kidney disease. A useful alternative, however, is to use spectacles that cut out the blue component of light. Worn in the evening, these will stimulate the production of natural melatonin, which has no harmful side effects.

REFLEXOLOGY

Reflexology is a form of foot massage whose theory is based on the belief that the whole of the body is reflected in microcosm in the foot. In other words, massage of one area of the foot will affect the lungs, another the thyroid gland, a third the intestines and so on. The treatment itself is extremely relaxing and has been used over the years to treat a wide range of conditions.

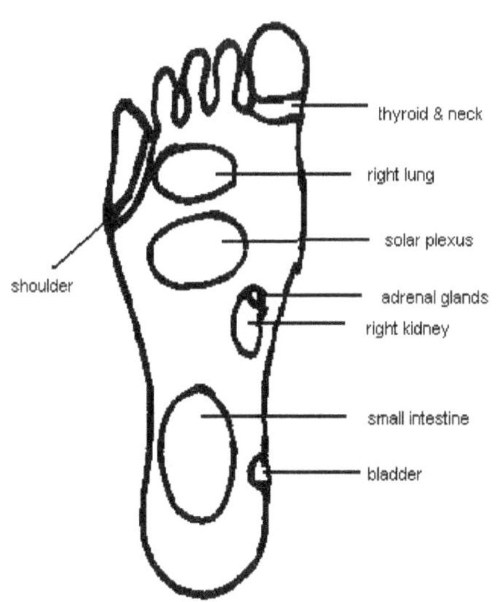

Some of the reflex areas on the right foot

A study carried out in China looked at the effect of reflexology on 70 patients suffering from insomnia. They were divided into two groups, the first being given 20 minutes of reflexology twice a day for ten days and the second having 20 minutes once a day over the same period. Over half these patients had had insomnia for more than three years and over a third were dependent on sleeping pills. Despite this, after 10 days of treatment all those in the first group reported that they were now sleeping naturally, without pills, and were feeling relaxed and clear minded during the day. However, only a quarter of those in the second group were able to say this. It would seem, on the basis of this study, that if you were to consider having some reflexology treatment for your insomnia, you would have to be prepared for a considerable number of treatments. It may be, of course, that you could find a therapist who would show you how to treat yourself so that you could massage your feet twice daily between treatment sessions and thus speed up your recovery.

SHIATSU

Shiatsu is a Japanese therapy whose theory is not unlike that of acupuncture, with the idea of energy being carried around the body in a series of channels or meridians. The aim of the treatment, like that of acupuncture, is to restore the flow of energy to normal and, as a result, restore the body to normal function.

Various techniques are used, including pressure on the relevant points, as well as more vigorous stretching and rotating of joints. Usually the treatment is given on a padded mat on the floor, although patients who find this difficult can be treated sitting on a chair.

Although a full treatment from a qualified practitioner is preferable, there are points that you can try using yourself before bedtime, pressing gently but firmly with your thumb:

- to the side of each eye, between the eyebrow and the outer corner of the eye, about one finger's width away from the end of the eyebrow: press for 7 to 10 seconds.

- on the sole of the foot about a third of the distance along a line running from the tip of the middle toe to the heel: press for 10 to 15 seconds.

- about an inch and a half to each side of the spine, at the level of the upper edge of the hip bones: press for 5 to 7 seconds and repeat twice more.

- midway along a line running across the top of the head between the upper tips of the ears: press down with both thumbs for 10 to 15 seconds.

TRADITIONAL CHINESE MEDICINE

The theory underlying TCM is the same as that of acupuncture and diagnosis is made in the same way, using the pulse and tongue. However, whereas acupuncture uses needles to restore Qi to normal, TCM uses herbs.

According to TCM, there are a number of different types of insomnia, each of which is treated with different herbs or herbal mixtures.

The types of insomnia include:

- difficulty falling asleep followed by action-filled dreams or nightmares; irritability or anxiety during the day, a dry mouth with a bitter taste, constipation, headache and dizziness. A red tongue with a yellow coating and a wiry rapid pulse will confirm the diagnosis of stagnation of Qi causing Heat in the Liver.

- similar symptoms associated with a yellow greasy coating on the tongue and a rapid slippery pulse is likely to be diagnosed as the Heart being invaded by Heat and Phlegm.

- frequent waking during the night in an anxious state, absentmindedness and daydreaming, a pale tongue with a thin white coating and a thready pulse may be diagnosed as deficiency of Qi and Heart Blood.

- long-standing insomnia associated with vivid dreams, worry and fear, dizziness, a poor memory, weakness in the back and knees and night sweating may be due to a Heart and Kidney disharmony and would be confirmed by a red tongue with a scanty yellow coating and a thready, rapid pulse.

As you can see, different types of insomnia may share similar symptoms and, although you can probably work out from your symptoms which type of insomnia you *might* be suffering from, it needs a qualified practitioner to confirm this by pulse and tongue diagnosis. Unlike some other types of complementary medicine, such as homeopathy, if you take the wrong herbs, there is a risk that you will make yourself worse and not better. So, for this reason, it's not a good idea to use TCM as a self-help treatment but, rather, to consult a qualified practitioner.

YOGA

A brief introduction

Scientific trials, including one carried out in England involving 3000 yoga students, have shown that practicing yoga can help you sleep better. While yoga can have very beneficial effects on both body and mind, there are some conditions which make certain postures inadvisable. If you are in any doubt, consult your physician before trying any yoga exercises.

Several postures, such as Adho Mukha Svanasana (the Downward Facing Dog), Halasana (the Plow), Janu Sirsasana (the Knee Head Bend), Paschimottanasana (the Great Western Stretch), Salamba Sarvangasana (the Supported Shoulder Stand), Salamba Sirsasana (the Supported Head Stand), Setu Bandha Sarvangasana (the Bridge) and Uttanasana (the Great Stretch), are said to be specifically beneficial for people who suffer from insomnia but because the benefits will only be apparent if you perform them correctly, you really need to go to a class rather than try to learn the exercises out of a book. In addition, postures do not stand alone but are usually performed in sequences which are best learned from a qualified teacher.

However, there is one posture – Shavasana or the Corpse – which can be learned from a book and performed safely without a teacher.

The Corpse Posture (Shavasana)

Although this may sound easy – little more than lying on your back, you may think – it's harder than it appears. It needs to be practiced for not less than 15 minutes at least twice a day if you are to reap any benefits. If you can spare the time, you can stay in the posture for up to an hour. Because you can become very deeply relaxed while practicing Shavasana, you need to make certain that you're not going to be disturbed. Unplug the 'phone and hang a "do not disturb" sign on your door. When you decide you've had enough, come out of the posture very slowly.

Lie on your back on the floor (use a thick rug or mat to make yourself more comfortable) with your feet about six inches apart and your toes pointing outwards. Let your arms lie at a slight angle so your hands are a few inches from your body, palm up. Relax your fingers. Turn your head slightly to the right or left and shut your eyes.

Stay like this, not moving at all, for a few minutes. Breathe normally and try just to be aware of your body. Then, starting at the top of your head and working slowly downwards, concentrate on allowing each group of muscles to relax in turn – the scalp, the forehead, the face, the chin, the neck and so on all the way down to your toes. Once you have done this, remain still and comfortable for as long as you wish.

CONCLUSION

I hope that somewhere among all these different therapies and treatments you will find something to help you. When you try one, be patient – give it time to work. If you feel even the slightest improvement after a week or two, then persevere. It may take weeks or even months before you're sleeping completely normally again, particularly if you've been an insomniac for a long time. But keep the end result in mind and don't give up hope.

If a therapy gives some relief but doesn't seem as though it's going to do any more than that, try combining it with something else. Usually this isn't a problem although you shouldn't combine orthodox medicine with any form of herbal treatment (because they may interact) or with homeopathy (because drugs make it difficult for homeopathic remedies to work). If you're being treated by a therapist, always check with them before adding another therapy. It may take time but, sooner or later, (and hopefully sooner) you should find a therapy or therapies that suit you. And when you do, stick with them.

I wish you good health, peaceful nights and sweet dreams.

RESOURCES

These are just a few of the many creators and suppliers of remedies. For more information on what is available, try searching online for 'flower remedies', 'crystal essences' or 'homeopathic remedies'.

FLOWER REMEDIES

Australian bush flower essences

http://ausflowers.com.au

Tel: +61 2 9450 1388

Alaskan flower essences

https://www.alaskanessences.com/

Orders: +1 800-545-9309 (N.America)

Customer Service: +1 406-642-3670

Spirit-in-Nature essences

http://spirit-in-nature.com/

Tel: +1 800.347.3639

+1 530.478.7655

Pacific essences

https://www.pacificessences.com/

Tel: +1-250-384-5560

Fax: +1-250-595-7700

Living essences of Australia

http://livingessences.com.au/

+61 (0)8 93011234

Tree Frog Farm flower essences

http://www.treefrogfarm.com/

Tel: +1 (360) 758-7260

BACH FLOWER REMEDIES

The Bach Centre

http://www.bachcentre.com/index.php

+44 (0)1491 834678

CRYSTAL ESSENCES

Crystal Herbs

http://www.crystalherbs.com/

+44 1379 608059

HOMEOPATHIC REMEDIES

Helios Pharmacy

http://www.helios.co.uk/

+44 (0)1892 537254

+44 (0)1892 536393 (24 hours)

INDEX

www.ingramcontent.com/pod-product-compliance
Lightning Source LLC
Chambersburg PA
CBHW061513050726
47593CB00002B/545